# Ultrasound Guided Procedures and Radiologic Imaging for Pediatric Anesthesiologists

**ANESTHESIA ILLUSTRATED**
Keith J. Ruskin, MD and Barbara K. Burian, PhD
Series Editors

**Published and Forthcoming Titles:**

*Pediatric Anesthesia Procedures*, edited by Anna Clebone and Barbara K. Burian

*Ultrasound Guided Procedures and Radiologic Imaging for Pediatric Anesthesiologists*, edited by Anna Clebone, Joshua H. Finkle, and Barbara K. Burian

*Emergency Anesthesia Procedures*, edited by Lauren Berkow

*Cancer Pain Procedures*, edited by Amit Gulati

*Radiologic Imaging for the Anesthesiologist*, edited by Keith Ruskin and Abraham Dachman

# Ultrasound Guided Procedures and Radiologic Imaging for Pediatric Anesthesiologists

**EDITED BY**

**Anna Clebone, MD**
Associate Professor
Department of Anesthesia and Critical Care
The University of Chicago
Chicago, IL

**Joshua H. Finkle, MD**
Pediatric Radiology
Advocate Children's Hospital
Park Ridge, IL

**Barbara K. Burian, PhD**
Human Systems Integration Division
NASA Ames Research Center
Moffett Field, CA

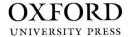

OXFORD
UNIVERSITY PRESS

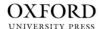

Oxford University Press is a department of the University of Oxford. It furthers
the University's objective of excellence in research, scholarship, and education
by publishing worldwide. Oxford is a registered trade mark of Oxford University
Press in the UK and certain other countries.

Published in the United States of America by Oxford University Press
198 Madison Avenue, New York, NY 10016, United States of America.

Library of Congress Cataloging-in-Publication Data
Names: Clebone, Anna, editor. | Finkle, Joshua H., editor. | Burian, Barbara K., editor.
Title: Ultrasound guided procedures and radiologic imaging for pediatric anesthesiologists /
edited by Anna Clebone, Joshua H. Finkle, Barbara K. Burian.
Description: New York, NY : Oxford University Press, [2021] |
Includes bibliographical references and index.
Identifiers: LCCN 2021006072 (print) | LCCN 2021006073 (ebook) | ISBN 9780190081416 (paperback) |
ISBN 9780190081430 (epub) | ISBN 9780190081447
Subjects: MESH: Anesthesia | Child | Surgery, Computer-Assisted—methods | Ultrasonography—methods
Classification: LCC RD139 (print) | LCC RD139 (ebook) | NLM WO 440 | DDC 617.9/6083—dc23
LC record available at https://lccn.loc.gov/2021006072
LC ebook record available at https://lccn.loc.gov/2021006073

DOI: 10.1093/med/9780190081416.001.0001

9 8 7 6 5 4 3 2 1

Printed by Integrated Books International, United States of America

# Contents

## PART IV: RADIOLOGY

# Preface

Procedures in pediatric anesthesiology were historically taught using actual patients, with little or no student preparation. In recent years, this has rightfully become unacceptable. The side effect, however, is that the performance of such procedures is pushed to later in training, with clinicians having fewer opportunities to perform them before independent practice. Simulations, including part-task trainers, have been used with some success; however, these sessions are often limited and, by nature, may not include the repetition or variation in presentation needed for learning and deep understanding.

In traditional textbooks, procedures are typically described at length, with much attention given to research findings that may have little direct or clear relevance to how a procedure actually ought to be carried out. Additionally, the lengthy paragraphs in which they are written do not readily translate into actual guidance for procedure execution. Furthermore, they are naturally restricted in the number of illustrations provided and may be narrow in the procedural skills described.

In this text, we address these shortcomings by providing well-illustrated and clearly defined and actionable guidance. This guide is intended as a ready resource for both experts and novices. It will be useful to those with extensive training and experience as well as beginners and those with remote experience and training. A wealth of knowledge in the human factors of procedure design and use has been applied throughout to ensure that desired information can be easily located, that steps are clearly identified and comprehensible, and that additional information of high relevance to procedure completion is co-located and salient.

This book begins with the basics but quickly progresses to advanced skill sets. It is divided into four parts. Part I starts with a primer on ultrasound machine functionality as well as procedural chapters on lung ultrasound to detect a mainstem intubation or pneumothorax and gastric ultrasound to assess gastric contents in incompletely fasted patients. Part II covers ultrasound guided peripheral intravenous line placement through the incremental advancement method, ultrasound guided arterial line placement, and ultrasound guided central line placement. Part III details several ultrasound guided regional anesthesia techniques. Part IV covers radiology of the pediatric airway and mediastinum, lungs, gastrointestinal, genitourinary, musculoskeletal, and neurologic systems.

Another book serves as a companion volume to this one and is titled *Pediatric Anesthesia Procedures*. This companion book includes a primer on airway and breathing functionality as well as procedural chapters on specialty skills such as lung isolation. It continues on to cover vascular access, from the fundamentals of fluid management and programming several types of common pumps to intraosseous placement. Neuraxial regional anesthesia techniques are also detailed, as are sympathetic blocks performed by those with an additional fellowship in pain management. *Pediatric Anesthesia Procedures* concludes with emergencies and critical conditions, including cardiopulmonary resuscitation for neonates and older children and treatment of local anesthetic systemic toxicity. It also includes four chapters that detail the anesthetic management for classic neonatal surgical pathologies, such as tracheoesophageal fistula, myelomeningocele, gastroschisis/omphalocele, and congenital diaphragmatic hernia.

We hope that these volumes will serve as a guide for both beginners and experts to pediatric anesthesiology procedures and will benefit children everywhere.

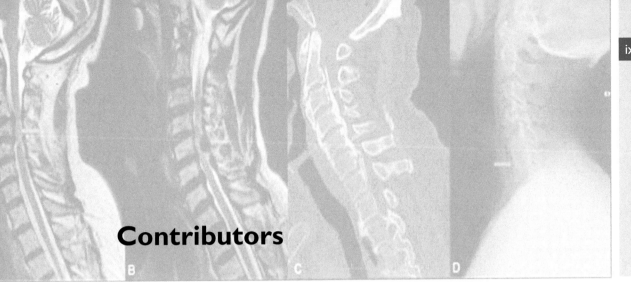

# Contributors

**Hubert A. Benzon, MD, MPH, FAAP**
Associate Professor of Anesthesiology
Pediatric Anesthesiology, Ann & Robert H. Lurie
Children's Hospital of Chicago
Northwestern University Feinberg School of Medicine
Chicago, IL

**Brooke Albright-Trainer, MD**
Assistant Professor of Anesthesiology
Department of Anesthesiology and Critical Care
Medicine
Central Virginia VA Health Care System
Virginia Commonwealth University
Richmond, VA

**Barbara K. Burian, PhD**
Senior Research Psychologist
Human Systems Integration Division
NASA Ames Research Center
Moffett Field, CA

**Anna Clebone, MD**
Associate Professor
Department of Anesthesia and Critical Care
The University of Chicago
Chicago, IL

**Joshua H. Finkle, MD**
Pediatric Radiology
Advocate Children's Hospital
Park Ridge, IL

**Nicholas Florence, MD**
Resident Physician
Diagnostic Radiology
University of Chicago Medicine
Chicago, IL

**Christopher Johnson, MD**
Chicago, IL

**Natalea Johnson, MD**
Pediatric Anesthesiologist
Oregon Anesthesiology Group
Providence St. Vincent's Medical Center
Portland, OR

**Mohammed Mohsin Khadir, MD**
Interventional Radiologist
Munster Radiology Group
Community Hospital
Munster, Indiana

**Michael R. King, MD**
Assistant Professor of Anesthesiology
Pediatric Anesthesiology, Ann & Robert H. Lurie
Children's Hospital of Chicago and Northwestern
University Feinberg School of Medicine
Chicago, IL

**Ramesh Kodavatiganti, MD, FASA**
Assistant Professor of Anesthesiology
Department of Anesthesiology and Critical Care,
Division of Cardiac Anesthesia, Children's Hospital of
Philadelphia and University of Pennsylvania Perelman
School of Medicine
Philadelphia, PA

**Kirk Lalwani, MD, FRCA, MCR**
Professor of Anesthesiology and Pediatrics
Vice-Chair for Faculty Development
Director, Pediatric Anesthesiology Fellowship Program
Anesthesiology, BTE-2
Oregon Health and Science University
Portland, OR

**Ann F. T. Lawrence, DO**
Associate Professor of Anesthesiology and Pediatrics
Division Chief of Pediatric Anesthesiology, The
University of Vermont Medical Center
The University of Vermont Larner College of Medicine
Burlington, VT

**Jorge A. Pineda, MD**
Associate Professor
Pediatric Anesthesiology, Doernbecher Children's
Hospital
Oregon Health & Science University School of
Medicine
Portland, OR

**Syed Ali Raza, MD**
Anesthesiology Resident
Department of Anesthesia and Critical Care
University of Chicago Medicine
Chicago, IL

**J. Devin Roberts, MD**
Clinical Instructor
Department of Anesthesiology,
Critical Care and Pain Medicine
NorthShore University Health System
Chicago, IL

**Corey Sheahan, MD**
Clinical Instructor and Chronic Pain Fellow
University of Vermont Medical Center
The University of Vermont Larner College
of Medicine
Burlington, VT

**Philip W. Yun, DO**
Assistant Professor of Anesthesiology
Pediatric Anesthesiology, Doernbecher Children's
Hospital
Oregon Health & Science University
Portland, OR

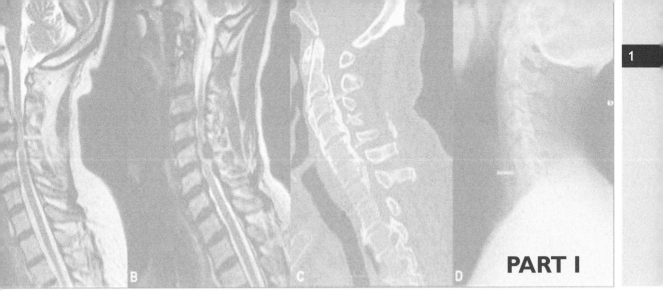

**PART I**

# BASIC ULTRASOUND
# PROCEDURES

# Chapter 1

# Ultrasound Physics and Ultrasound Machine Functionality

*Brooke Albright-Trainer*

# Basic Physics and Concepts of Ultrasound

The human ear can appreciate sounds between the frequencies of 20 and 20,000 Hz. At more than 20,000 Hz, the frequency is considered "ultrasound." Frequency is defined as the number of cycles over a period of time and is measured in Hertz (cycles/second). Ultrasound is a form of energy transmitted as cyclic oscillations through mediums, such as the human body, and its velocity is constant. The velocity of sound is equal to wavelength multiplied by frequency. All ultrasound waves are characterized by a specific wavelength and frequency. Because velocity is constant, if the frequency increases, the wavelength must decrease, and vice versa. In terms of distance, the higher the frequency, the shorter distance a sound wave travels (Figure 1.1). This concept is at the core of ultrasound guided regional anesthesia because different frequency probes are used for different blocks.

Ultrasound medical imaging (also known as sonography) is a diagnostic imaging tool that uses high-frequency sound waves to create images of structures in the body. Ultrasound can show details that a still image like an X-ray cannot, such as blood flow or needle guidance to a nerve. A lower frequency (larger wavelength) ultrasound wave will penetrate deeper but will lack the resolution (ability to delineate between two or more points/objects in space) of the higher frequency and smaller wavelength beam. Ultrasound images are captured in real time using an external transducer probe directly on the skin. The transducer utilizes electrical energy (alternating current) and turns it into sound energy when the signal is placed across piezoelectric crystals, causing them to vibrate through the body. These ultrasound waves travel into the body and are reflected off of objects, returning some of the energy as mechanical energy back to the transducer. When this mechanical energy strikes the transducer, the crystals vibrate, again converting the energy back into electrical energy, which is translated by computer software and displayed on a screen (Figure 1.2).

By convention, the more mechanical energy that is reflected back to the transducer and converted, the whiter or more echogenic the structure will appear. Ultrasound waves lose energy as they travel through tissue, largely as a result of a viscoelastic absorption process. The more energy that is refracted or attenuated (absorbed) and not converted, the darker the image appears. In this way, the physician is able to identify structures and pathological conditions by distinguishing different shades of gray (Figure 1.3). Usually, at a given distance, a lower frequency wave will attenuate less than a higher frequency wave. Therefore, deeper penetration into the tissue is achieved with a lower frequency ultrasound wave.

Cardiac imaging is a good example of a clear demarcation between ultrasound wave reflection, refraction, and attenuation (Figure 1.4). The myocardium reflects more waves and thus appears whiter (hyperechoic), and the blood-filled chambers absorb (attenuate) and/or refract many of the waves, thus appearing darker (hypoechoic or anechoic). For regional anesthesia,

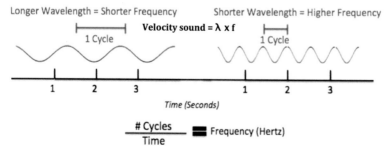

**Figure 1.1** Understanding the relationship between wavelength and frequency (Hertz).

Wall electricity/battery -> Electrical energy -> Ultrasound -> Mechanical energy -> Electrical energy

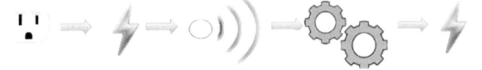

Figure 1.2  How ultrasound energy is created and converted into translatable information.

## Gray-White Composition

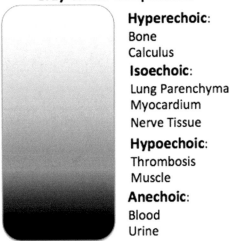

**Hyperechoic**:
Bone
Calculus
**Isoechoic**:
Lung Parenchyma
Myocardium
Nerve Tissue
**Hypoechoic**:
Thrombosis
Muscle
**Anechoic**:
Blood
Urine

Figure 1.3  Distinguishing shades of gray in ultrasound images.

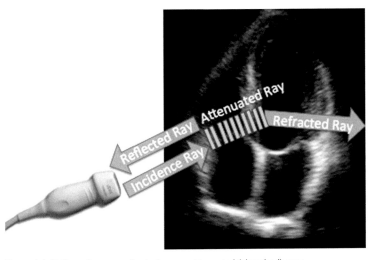

Figure 1.4  Reflected versus refracted versus attenuated (absorbed) rays.

it can be challenging to make a positive identification of a structure on ultrasound because nerves and muscles will often have a similar appearance. In other words, there is a lack of a clear acoustic interface between these structures.

So far, there is no firm evidence of a biohazard from diagnostic ultrasound use in humans. Most biohazards discussed are theoretical or are only seen in animal models in extreme or unusual situations. The greatest heating of tissue is typically associated with multiple pulsing modes such as Doppler imaging and high-frame-rate, high-line-density modes. At typical levels of exposure and intensities, ultrasound is able to raise the local temperature of tissues by a few degrees Celsius; however, this has been shown to be clinically insignificant.

## Understanding the Ultrasound Machine and Its Components

The ultrasound machine is best understood if it is broken down into its various parts and modalities. Keep in mind that not all ultrasound machines have the same functions. Some machines are better equipped for specific tasks, such as echocardiography, which requires more precise measurements of the heart and calculations of blood flow. Figure 1.5 is an example of an ultrasound machine commonly used for regional anesthesia.

You will notice that this ultrasound machine lacks the ability to apply focus, time gain compensation (TGC), or continuous or pulsed wave Doppler. On this machine, the functions have been simplified for everyday use, such as in regional anesthesia.

## "Knobology": Ultrasound Machine Knobs and Their Functions

### Machine Operation

- **Power:** Turns device on or off
- **Soft keys:** Six sets of two-button controls adjust the values of each control displayed in the context menu; vary depending on mode or feature activated

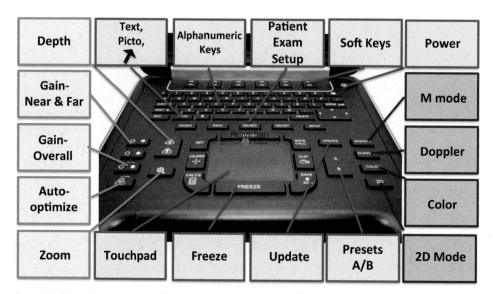

Figure 1.5 Selected ultrasound machine buttons. Labels for ultrasound operating modes are in purple, and labels for ultrasound image optimization are in green.

- **Patient exam setup keys:** Access the patient information, display system settings, review patient lists, save images, archive, open exam menu
- **Save calc:** Saves calculations and measurements and transfers to patient report
- **Alphanumeric keys:** Used to enter text and numbers
- **Exam:** Switch between different exam types, e.g., nerve, vascular, musculoskeletal (Msk)
- **Set:** Confirms caliper location for measurements
- **Text:** Turns the alphanumeric keyboard on/off for text entry
- **Picto:** Turns the pictograph marker on/off
- **Caliper:** Activates up to eight different calipers on the screen
- **Calc:** Turns the calculation menu on/off
- **Select/touchpad:** These are used together to make various choices, depending on function toggled. Select items on screen (e.g., switch between color and Doppler options, arrow position and orientation, calipers for measurement). Touchpad adjusts and moves items on screen.
- **Freeze:** Stops live image, displays frozen image
- **Save:** Allows you to save an image of the structure to internal storage of the system
- **Clip:** Allows you to save a movie of the image from 2 to 60 seconds
- **Update:** Allows toggling between dual and duplex screens in image modes, M-mode, and Doppler
- **Presets (A/B):** Parameter or shortcut, programmable keys that can be chosen from a dropdown menu to perform common tasks
- **Arrow:** Turns on an arrow, which can be moved and rotated within an image area

### Ultrasound Operating Modes

Different modes are used primarily for assessment of fluid motion and flow. Use these to confirm or differentiate between vascular structures.

- **M-mode:** Turns M-mode on/off and toggles between sample line and trace
- **Doppler:** Turns Doppler on/off and toggles between sample line and trace
- **Color:** This button turns color or color power Doppler on/off (Figure 1.6), which provides a two-dimensional (2D) view of blood flow in real time displayed in full color, with various

**Top Color:**
Flow toward
the transducer

**No Doppler shift
at 90-degree angle**

**Bottom Color:**
Flow away from
the transducer

**Figure 1.6** Color flow Doppler diagram.

colors representing both positive and negative velocities, depending on the direction of blood flow to the transducer. This function is helpful when differentiating vascular structures. The top color (i.e., red) indicates flow toward the transducer, and the bottom color (i.e., blue) indicates flow away from the transducer.

- **Duplex:** Color Doppler on top of gray-scale B mode
- **Pulsed wave (PW)** and **continuous wave (CW):** Pulsed wave is a Doppler recording of blood flow velocities in a range-specific area along the length of the beam. Continuous wave is a Doppler recording of blood flow velocities along the length of the beam. These functions are most useful in cardiac exams and are rarely, if ever, used in ultrasound guided regional anesthesia.
- **2D Mode:** This is the scanning mode that is normally used. A 2D cross-sectional view is used for locating and measuring anatomical structures and for spatial orientation in real time. Ultrasound waves of different lengths and intensities are displayed in up to 256 gray shades.
- **Needle guidance:** The machine can display a pair of guidance lines to represent the anticipated path of the needle. These lines overlay the 2D image of the anatomical target. This feature depends on the transducer and exam type.

## Ultrasound Image Optimization

When images are difficult to obtain, knowledge of a few knob functions will help the operator optimize the image. One technique is to adjust the relevant knobs, in the following sequential order:

1. **Depth:** Depth determines how long the ultrasound machine will listen for returning signals. The ideal point of interest should be in the middle of the screen to optimally characterize necessary structures and adjust as needed throughout the scan. Start "deeper" and decrease depth to put the area of interest either in the middle of the screen or at three-fourths of the depth of the screen.

2. **Focus:** Focus provides an improved resolution of a particular depth at the focal points. Place focal points at region of interest. Modern machines have multiple focal zones. When the number of focal zones is increased, the frame rate is decreased.

3. **Zoom:** Magnify point of interest.

4. **Gain:** Gain refers to the amplification of the received signal. This determines the brightness of the image, and optimal gain allows for proper distinction of structures. Of note, most beginners use gain that is too high, which can obscure many details.

5. **TGC (near, far):** TGC compensates for beam attenuation. This allows you to vary the gain according to your depth. For instance, you may have a bright structure in the near field but want to see a structure in the far field. You can preferentially turn down gain in the far and near fields independently. This helps obtain a smooth gray-scale picture.

6. **Dynamic range:** Dynamic range allows you to adjust for the contrast (i.e., how white is white, how black is black?)—settings include −3, −2, −1, 0, +1, +2, +3. Negative numbers show higher contrast images (decreased number of grays displayed), and positive numbers show low contrast (increased number of grays).

7. **Auto-optimize:** Auto-optimize adds more contrast to the image—whites are whiter, blacks are blacker. It must be deselected and then reselected for every new structure imaged.

# Transducer Probes

Transducer probes are available in different sizes and shapes, each optimized for different purposes. Most transducers used for ultrasound guided regional anesthesia operate between 4 and 13 million Hz (megahertz [MHz]). Some of the most common transducer probes are:

- **Linear array transducer probe** (7.5 MHz; 13–6 MHz, 25 mm; 10–5 MHz, 38 mm) (Figure 1.7): Rectangular field of view, piezoelectric elements arranged in parallel sequentially activated to produce an image, less loss of resolution with depth, useful to scan superficial structures with high frequency, such as for vascular access or for peripheral nerves

- **Phased array transducer probe** (5–1 MHz, 21 mm): Smaller scanning surface, more narrow footprint, same loss of resolution with depth as linear array probe, useful for echocardiography, more expensive, elements activated with phase differences to allow steering of the ultrasound signal

- **Curved array transducer probe** (5–2 MHz, 11 mm; 5–2 MHz, 60 mm) (Figure 1.7): Large scanning area, loss of resolution with depth, better penetration, useful in abdominal/pelvic scans such as in obstetrics or for the focused assessment with sonography in trauma (FAST) exam

- **Sector transducer probe:** Pie-shaped field of view—resolution poorer at increasing depth
  Acoustic coupling gel must be used during exams between the transducer and the body to obtain suitable images. For invasive or sterile use, a transducer sheath may be used along with a liberal amount of sterile gel. Structures of interest can be imaged either in the short axis (cross section) or the long axis. A short-axis view becomes a long-axis view when the transducer is turned 90 degrees in either direction. In general, regional anesthesiologists prefer to image nerves and blood vessels in the short axis. This is because the short axis gives the operator a simultaneous anterior-posterior and lateral-medial perspective. In the long-axis view, the lateral-medial perspective is lost.

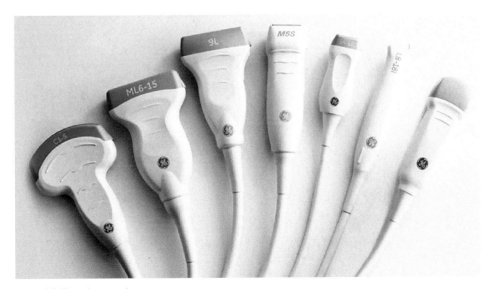

Figure 1.7 Transducer probes.

# Conclusion

Several tools and techniques are useful in acquiring the best ultrasound image. First and foremost, it is important that ultrasound users learn sonographic anatomy. Second, clinicians must learn to use the correct ultrasound machine and transducer to obtain the best image for the point of interest. Third, clinicians must master the knobs of the machine in order to optimize the image. For example, gain must be maximized before increasing power. TGC should be smooth. It is better to go from a wider field of view and zoom in, and it is better to start deeper and then adjust the image to be more shallow. Clinicians should also acquire images in at least two planes. To prevent infection, remember to wipe off and disinfect the transducer after every use and to wear gloves, even on the scanning hand. Clinicians must also learn proper maintenance of the machine and transducers and remember to switch off the machine after use, "freeze" when not scanning, handle with care, clean with a soft towel, and disinfect after every use.

# Further Readings

Sites BD, Chan VW, Neal JM, et al. The American Society of Regional Anesthesia and Pain Medicine and the European Society of Regional Anaesthesia and Pain Therapy Joint Committee Recommendations for Education and Training in Ultrasound-Guided Regional Anesthesia. *Reg Anethes Pain Med*. 2009;34:40–46.

*SonoSite Manual*. Available at: https://www.sonosite.com/support/documents.

# Chapter 2

# Lung Ultrasound to Detect Pneumothorax or Mainstem Intubation

*J. Devin Roberts and Anna Clebone*

# Introduction

In healthy patients, a layer of visceral pleura will slide on the parietal pleura with every breath. This can be readily imaged with a handheld ultrasound probe at the point of care, and this information can be used for diagnosis of pneumothorax or mainstem intubation. Lung ultrasound can also help the clinician to visualize pleural effusions or pulmonary edema.[1] When trying to diagnose pneumothorax by imaging, lung ultrasound is more accurate for ruling pneumothorax in (level B evidence) or out (level A evidence) than supine anterior chest radiograph.[2]

# Clinical Applications

| **WARNING!!** | Lung sliding may not occur if the patient has acute respiratory distress syndrome or lung fibrosis, is having an acute asthma attack, or has undergone a pleurodesis in the past, because the visceral and parietal pleura may be adherent to each other. |
|---|---|

Visualizing lung sliding with ultrasound will rule out pneumothorax at the point of the lung that is being imaged and will rule out a mainstem intubation (100% positive predictive value for both). In one study in which the endotracheal tube was deliberately placed in either the trachea or a mainstem bronchus under fiberoptic guidance, "identification of tracheal *versus* bronchial intubation was 62% (26 of 42) in the auscultation group and 95% (40 of 42) in the ultrasound group" by using lung ultrasound to look for pleural lung sliding.[3] Identifying a mainstem intubation may be even more important in pediatric patients than in adult patients: "The American Society of Anesthesiologists Closed Claims Project showed that bronchial intubation accounts for 2% of adverse respiratory claims in adults and 4% in children."[3]

# Contraindications

An open wound over the ultrasound site may be a contraindication. A sterile ultrasound probe cover must be used if lung ultrasound is performed in a sterile field.

# Critical Anatomy

We suggest taking a systematic approach by dividing the chest into four quadrants, which will allow you to examine common pathology[2] (Figure 2.1).

# Setup

## Equipment

- Ultrasound machine
- High-frequency 3- to 5-MHz probe
- Ultrasound gel
- Sterile ultrasound probe cover and sterile gel if performing ultrasound on a sterile field

# Step-by-Step

1. **Position the patient.** The patient may be in any position but typically is placed supine.
2. **Place the ultrasound probe.** Place the ultrasound probe longitudinally on the chest in the second intercostal space, with the probe marker pointing toward the head of the patient. Slide the ultrasound probe downward until you obtain a good view of the pleura (Figure 2.2).

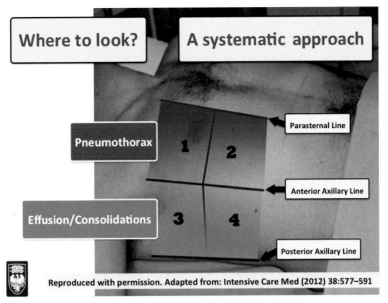

Figure 2.1 A systematic approach to lung ultrasound, dividing the chest into four quadrants to examine
common lung pathology.

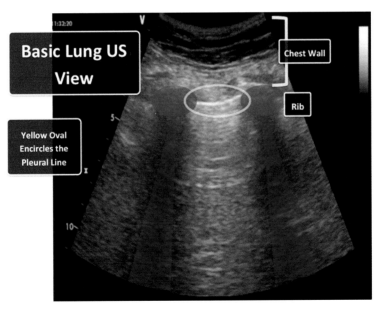

Figure 2.2 Basic ultrasound view.

> **WARNING!!** When imaging the left lung (or right lung if the patient has dextrocardia), the pericardium can be mistaken for the pleura; both are similar in appearance. The pericardium will move with each heartbeat.
>
> In some patients, the pleura itself will also slide slightly with each heartbeat, independent of respirations. Lung sliding that is a reflection of cardiac contraction will be at the rate of the heartbeat. Lung sliding due to respiration will be at the rate of breathing.

3. **Interpret the image.** Interpretation of lung ultrasound is largely based on interpreting artifactual aspects of the image. When the lungs are inflated, the air halts progression of the ultrasound beam; therefore, information is gathered from the artifacts that occur after the ultrasound beam is stopped. When interpreting lung ultrasound to detect a pneumothorax, look for lung sliding, the lung point, A lines, and B lines (Figure 2.3).

   **To Look for Lung Sliding:** First, look for the ribs, which will appear as two anechoic black circles. Connecting these two circles is a hyperechoic line, also known as the "pleural line," which is where the visceral and parietal pleura meet (Figure 2.4). During respiration, as the visceral and parietal pleura slide over each other, a shimmering, to-and-fro movement will occur at the pleural line. This is known as "lung sliding," and it signifies that the lung is being ventilated. The presence of lung sliding rules out pneumothorax in the area of the lung that is being imaged, with a 100% positive predictive value. When a pneumothorax or hemothorax exists, the visceral and parietal pleura will be pushed apart by air or blood. In these situations, the visceral and parietal pleura will be separated and cannot slide over each other, and therefore lung sliding will not be seen. The absence of lung sliding may also be due to apnea, mainstem intubation, bronchospasm, acute respiratory distress syndrome, fibrosis, or severe atelectasis. Absence of lung sliding may also occur in a patient who is post pleurodesis.

*Pearl:* Lung sliding may be absent at the apex, even in normal lungs.

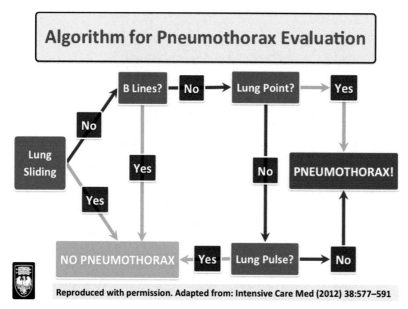

**Algorithm for Pneumothorax Evaluation**

Figure 2.3 Algorithm for pneumothorax evaluation.

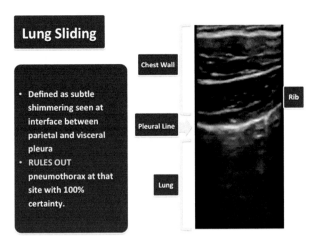

Figure 2.4 Lung sliding.

***Pearl:*** Lung sliding occurs in healthy patients of all ages and weights.

> **To Look for the Lung Point** (advanced technique)**:** The lung point can be difficult to find. It is the place where the pneumothorax starts (where the inflated lung and the pleural air meet); when found, the clinician will see both lung sliding and no lung sliding next to it in the same image.
>
> **To Look for A-Lines:** A-lines are seen because air causes the ultrasound beam to scatter. This scatter will appear as a regular, repeated, equidistant, motionless pattern of horizontal lines below the pleural line[4] (Figures 2.5 and 2.6). A-lines occur when the lung parenchyma

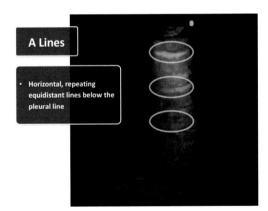

Figure 2.5 A lines.

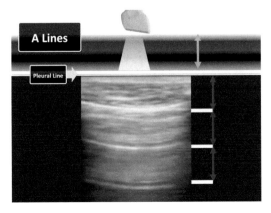

Figure 2.6 A lines.

(and therefore the air flowing through the lung) is not interrupted by lung injury (e.g., acute respiratory distress syndrome), blood, fluid (e.g., congestive heart failure pleural effusion), or pus (e.g., pneumonia)—all disease processes that are likely to show up on a chest radiograph. A helpful mnemonic is "**A**-line = normal **A**eration." When ventilation abnormalities occur, but A-lines are present, the ventilation abnormalities are more likely due to a cause unrelated to the lung parenchyma, such a pulmonary embolus or asthma.

**To Look for B-Lines (Lung Comets):** B-lines are hyperechoic rays which must start at the pleural line, move with the pleural line, and project vertically (Figures 2.7 and 2.8);

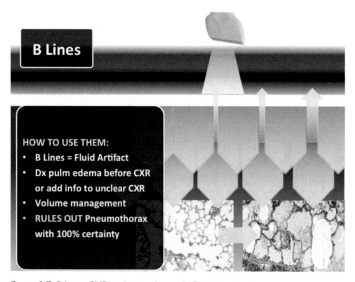

Figure 2.7  B lines. CXR = chest radiograph; Dx = diagnosis.

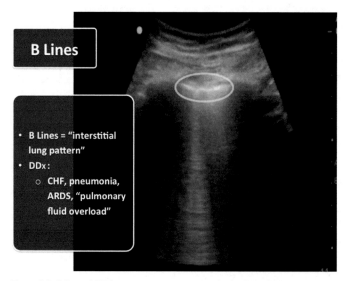

Figure 2.8  B lines. ARDS = acute respiratory distress syndrome; CHF = congestive heart failure; DDx = differential diagnosis.

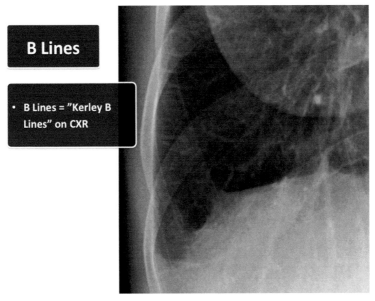

**B Lines**

- B Lines = "Kerley B Lines" on CXR

Figure 2.9 Kerley B lines on chest radiograph (CXR).

they are also known as "lung comets." Although one B-line can be normal, multiple B lines are an early sign of interstitial fluid (e.g., pulmonary edema) or thickening in the lungs. When more than one B-line is seen, this has similar implications as a ground-glass pattern on computed tomography scan or Kerley B lines on chest radiograph (Figure 2.9). The possible differential diagnosis for multiple B-lines includes pneumonia (early), congestive heart failure, interstitial lung disease, and acute respiratory distress syndrome. More B-lines may indicate more fluid. In one study, an increased number of lung comets was associated with increased severity of dyspnea, decreased ejection fraction, and increased diastolic dysfunction.[5,6] The presence of B-lines rules out pneumothorax with 100% certainty.

**Pearl:** B lines may be a more sensitive indicator of pulmonary edema than a chest radiograph.

## References

1. Lichtenstein DA, Meziere GA. Relevance of lung ultrasound in the diagnosis of acute respiratory failure: the BLUE protocol. *Chest.* 2008;134(1):117–125.
2. Volpicelli G, Elbarbary M, Blaivas M, et al. International evidence-based recommendations for point-of-care lung ultrasound. *Intensive Care Med.* 2012;38(4):577–591.
3. Ramsingh D, Frank E, Haughton R, et al. Auscultation versus point-of-care ultrasound to determine endotracheal versus bronchial intubation: a diagnostic accuracy study. *Anesthesiology.* 2016;124(5):1012–1020.

4. Lichtenstein DA, Meziere GA, Lagoueyte JF, et al. A-lines and B-lines: lung ultrasound as a bedside tool for predicting pulmonary artery occlusion pressure in the critically ill. *Chest.* 2009;136(4):1014–1020.
5. Picano E, Frassi F, Agricola E, et al. Ultrasound lung comets: a clinically useful sign of extravascular lung water. *J Am Soc Echocardiogr.* 2006 Mar;19(3):356–363.
6. Frassi F, Gargani L, Gligorova S, et al. Clinical and echocardiographic determinants of ultrasound lung comets. *Eur J Echocardiogr.* 2007;8(6):474–479.

Chapter 3

# Gastric Ultrasound and Assessment of Gastric Contents in Incompletely Fasted Patients

*Anna Clebone*

# Introduction

Although rare, aspiration of gastric contents can occur with general anesthesia or deep sedation. Factors associated with morbidity after aspiration include gastric contents that are solid or particulate matter, a volume of more than 0.8 mL/kg, and a pH of less than 2.5.

Gastric ultrasound can be used preoperatively to assess stomach contents. In one study in which 40 adults were randomized to either fast or ingest a standardized quantity of fluid/solid, gastric ultrasound had a positive predictive value of 0.98 and a negative predictive value of 1 for detecting gastric contents.[1] In children, a study of 200 fasted elective surgery patients showed that only two of these children had a gastric fluid volume correlating with a risk for aspiration.[2]

# Clinical Applications

In children, fasting status can be difficult to ascertain because children may have eaten on the morning of surgery without their parent's knowledge. In addition, children with disorders such as gastroparesis or incomplete gastric emptying may have increased stomach contents.

# Contraindications

Patient or parent refusal.

# Critical Anatomy

The antrum of the stomach is found between the anterior liver and the posterior pancreas. Five layers of the stomach exist, of which the easiest to see on ultrasound is the muscularis layer, which is echolucent.

# Setup

## Equipment
- Ultrasound machine
- Curvilinear 2- to 5-MHz abdominal ultrasound probe for larger children; 10- to 13-MHz linear high-frequency probe for smaller children
- Ultrasound gel

# Step-by-Step

1. **Position the patient.** Gastric ultrasound to assess stomach contents is performed in both the supine and right lateral decubitus positions.
2. **Place the ultrasound probe.** Place the ultrasound probe longitudinally on the stomach (Figure 3.1A and B). The goal is to see a sagittal cross section of the gastric antrum; the plane that is visualized will include the aorta and the left lobe of the liver.[2]
3. **Interpret the ultrasound image** (Figure 3.2A–C). An empty stomach will be small, and content will not be visible inside the stomach itself. Content that is homogenous, hypoechoic, and less than 1.5 mL/kg indicates clear gastric fluid and can be normally present in appropriately fasted patients. A full stomach is indicated by stomach contents that are homogenous and hyperechoic (thick fluid), heterogenous and mixed echogenicity (solid particulate), or a "frosted-glass pattern" (solid particulate).

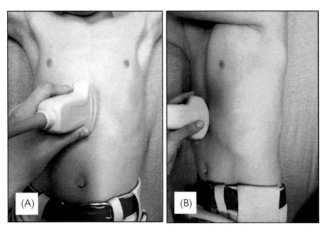

Figure 3.1 (**A** and **B**) Gastric ultrasound being performed in the epigastric location with a longitudinal ultrasound probe orientation. (Reproduced with permission from Leviter J, Steele DW, Constantine E, et al. Full
stomach despite the wait: point-of-care gastric ultrasound at the time of procedural sedation in the pediatric
emergency department. *Acad Emerg Med.* 2018 Oct 29 [Epub ahead of print], doi: 10.1111/acem.13651.)

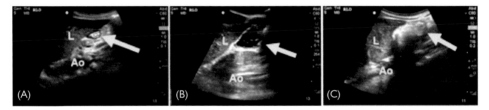

Figure 3.2 Gastric content seen on ultrasound in the epigastric location with a longitudinal ultrasound probe orientation. **A,** An empty gastric antrum looks flat, without content. **B,** Liquid gastric contents appear hypoechoic
or anechoic. **C,** Solid contents appear hyperechoic, often with a particulate appearance. Ao = aorta; L = liver;
*yellow arrow* = antrum. (Reproduced with permission from Leviter J, Steele DW, Constantine E, et al. Full stomach despite the wait: point-of-care gastric ultrasound at the time of procedural sedation in the pediatric emergency department. *Acad Emerg Med.* 2018 Oct 29 [Epub ahead of print], doi: 10.1111/acem.13651.)

4. **Calculate the volume of the gastric contents.**[2] The following formula was validated
   for children as young as 11 months of age:
   a. Between contractions of the antrum, determine the longitudinal diameter (D1) and the
      anterior-posterior diameter (D2) of the antrum, measuring from serosa to serosa.
   b. Calculate the antral area using the following formula:

   Antral area $= (\pi \times D1 \times D2)/4$

   c. Calculate the gastric content volume using the following formula:

   Volume (mL/kg) $= [-7.8 + 0.035 \times$ antral area measured in the right lateral decubitus
   $(mm^2) + 0.127 \times$ age (months)]/body weight (kg)

# References

1. Kruisselbrink R, Gharapetian A, Chaparro LE, et al. Diagnostic accuracy of point-of-care gastric ultrasound. *Anesth Analg*. 2019;128(1):89–95.
2. Bouvet L, Bellier N, Gagey-Riegel AC, et al. Ultrasound assessment of the prevalence of increased gastric contents and volume in elective pediatric patients: a prospective cohort study. *Paediatr Anaesth*. 2018;28(10):906–913.

PART II

# ULTRASOUND GUIDED VASCULAR ACCESS

## Chapter 4

# Ultrasound Guided Peripheral Intravenous Line Placement Using the Incremental Advancement Method

*Anna Clebone*

# Introduction

Ultrasound can be used to guide placement of multiple types of vascular access. In this chapter, I describe the dynamic use of ultrasound to guide the placement of a peripheral intravenous line, which leads to a high success rate.[1] In one prospective randomized study of pediatric patients younger than 10 years who underwent two previous unsuccessful attempts with standard techniques in the emergency department, the success rate increased by 16% with ultrasound guidance.[2] Skill with placing peripheral ultrasound guided intravenous lines in patients with difficult intravenous access can often help the practitioner avoid the need to place a central line (assuming the central line is not needed for other indications).[3]

# Clinical Applications

Ultrasound guided peripheral intravenous access is particularly useful in patients for whom there is difficulty with intravenous access.

# Contraindications

Contraindications for an intravenous line include an infection at the insertion site, limb compromise, an active dialysis fistula, prior lymph node dissection, or planned surgery on that limb. Special care should be taken at the median cubital site because this vein runs very close to the median nerve.

# Critical Anatomy

Arteries and veins are sonographically similar in cross section: hyperechoic circles with hypoechoic interiors. Arteries are more thickly walled and are characteristically pulsatile. Veins are more susceptible to compression. Doppler or color flow can distinguish amplitude and direction of flow. On color doppler, red indicates flow toward the transducer, and blue indicates flow away from the transducer (see Chapter 1). The presence of venous thrombosis is less likely in veins that are compressible.

# Setup

### Equipment

- Sterile prep, tourniquet, and an adhesive dressing
- Sterile gel—only a small amount is necessary
- Gauze—to wipe the gel off before engaging the Luer-Lok
- IV catheter/needles of assorted sizes and lengths, depending on the size and depth of the vein
- Local anesthetic (optional)—for a skin wheal in awake patients, typically use 0.5 to 1 mL of 1 to 2% lidocaine for local infiltration before puncturing the skin
- High-frequency linear ultrasound probe, 2 to 5 MHz, covered with a sterile occlusive dressing or sterile ultrasound probe cover (Figure 4.1)

# Step-by-Step

1. **Position the patient.** Stabilize the potential IV site. Towels and tape should be used to optimize the position of the limb. For example, placing a towel under the elbow to keep the elbow straight can assist with placing an antecubital IV line. For IV line placement into the cephalic vein, the clinician should partially supinate the arm to optimize the vein position, then use tape to stabilize the arm so that the arm remains in position during IV line placement.

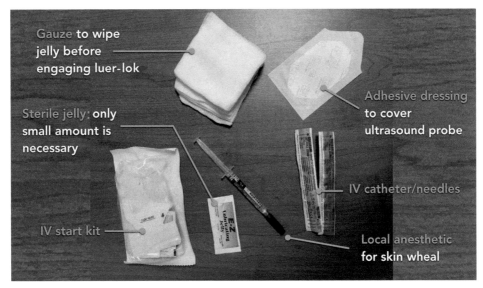

Gauze **to wipe jelly before engaging luer-lok**

**Sterile jelly: only small amount is necessary**

IV start kit

Adhesive dressing **to cover ultrasound probe**

IV catheter/needles

Local anesthetic **for skin wheal**

Figure 4.1 Equipment needed for ultrasound guided peripheral intravenous line placement.

>> **Tip on Technique:** Taking the time to ensure optimal positioning will greatly improve your success rate. It may be easier for the practitioner to sit while performing this procedure. Also, ensure that the ultrasound machine is placed so that the screen will be close to and directly in front of the practitioner and ensure that there is sufficient slack on the probe cord.

2. **Place the tourniquet and prep in a sterile fashion.** Place the tourniquet high on the limb so that you will have room to scan with the ultrasound probe. Prep widely to avoid contamination because you will be scanning up and down the arm with the ultrasound probe.

3. **Find a vein and then map it.** Ensure that the left side of the patient's limb corresponds with the left side of your ultrasound probe. Enable the guide line (line going down the center of the screen) on the ultrasound screen. After you have chosen a vein and optimized your ultrasound settings, carefully map the vein (Figure 4.2). Slide up and down the arm with the ultrasound probe to find an approach vector that is parallel to the vein. The probe should be aligned on an axis so that the vein remains in the center of the screen when the probe is moved proximally or distally for a distance corresponding to the entire length of your catheter. If the vein does not remain in the center of the screen (if you do not have a straight enough, long enough scan path), consider choosing a different location for cannulation (different section of the same vein, or different vein).

   In general, it is easier to cannulate a vein that is shallower and has a larger diameter. Change the ultrasound setting to the shallowest depth that will allow you to fully visualize the vein. Adjust the gain setting—in general, slightly less gain is more helpful for this procedure.

   >> **Tip on Technique:** It is important to ensure that you are cannulating a vein, not an artery. Veins are more compressible than arteries (however, arteries will compress as well, with enough pressure). Arteries may have a rounder appearance. There are two features on ultrasound imaging that may allow you to distinguish between an artery and a vein: color flow imaging, also called triplex ultrasound (which is a form of Doppler), and

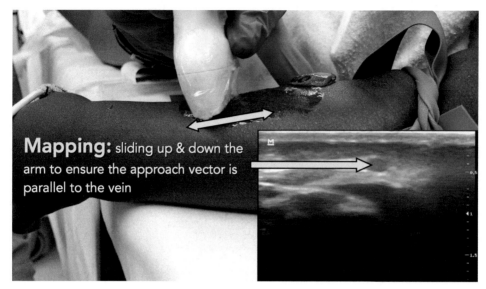

**Figure 4.2** Mapping the vein.

spectral Doppler. Pressing the "color" button will allow you to access color flow imaging, in which flow can be seen as either constant or pulsatile. Additionally, with color flow imaging, detected velocities are displayed as red or orange when blood is flowing toward the transducer and as blue when blood is flowing away from the transducer. For example, if the clinician is attempting to cannulate a vein and angles the probe in a distal direction (toward the hand), the artery will appear red and the vein will appear blue. On spectral Doppler, veins will have a flat waveform and arteries will have a peaked waveform.

>> **Tip on Technique:** Planting your fifth finger in a stable location as you scan up and down the arm can help you to stabilize your approach vector and consistently map it before and during the procedure.

>> **Tip on Technique:** The mid-forearm is often the best insertion site. Ideally, the entire length of the catheter will be below the elbow joint yet above the wrist joint. If the catheter crosses the joint, when the patient moves that joint, the IV line will not flow as well, and this movement will also increase the chance of infiltration. Additionally, catheters placed at or above the elbow joint may have a higher chance of thrombosis.

>> **Tip on Technique:** If a suitable scan path (straight, long enough, flow in the vein) is not immediately found, it is worthwhile to look at a variety of sites. It is often easiest to start at the antecubital fossa and scan distally at the following sites: median cubital vein (in the middle of the forearm), basilic vein (medial side of forearm), and cephalic vein (lateral side of forearm).

> **WARNING!!** Before cannulation, ensure that no contraindications to venous access for that limb/site exist (e.g., planned surgical procedure/graft, dialysis fistula, previous lymph node dissection).

> **WARNING!!** If the patient is likely to need semipermanent access (e.g., a periph-
> erally inserted central catheter (PICC) line) in the near future, avoid
> placing an intravenous line in the potential PICC site to avoid vessel
> damage.

4. **Choose a catheter size.** Using the ruler that is on the border of the ultrasound image, estimate the size of your vein and choose a catheter that is long enough that a sufficient portion of the catheter (at least one third of the catheter, ideally more) will lie intravascularly when the procedure is complete. The chosen catheter should also be a gauge that will fit into the vein (Table 4.1). When vein length will permit, choosing a longer catheter may lead to a longer lasting intravenous line; one recent study (in adults) showed that longer catheters had lower failure rates over time.[4] Using an IV catheter that is too short can lead to infiltration of the vein.

   >> **Tip on Technique:** For adult-sized pediatric patients, use a slightly longer standard IV catheter. Using a slightly longer catheter will potentially allow more of the catheter to be inserted into the vessel, decreasing the chance of infiltration.

   >> **Tip on Technique:** Before starting, loosen the catheter from the needle by advancing the catheter slightly off of the needle then returning the catheter to its original position. This is done so that the catheter will advance easily after blood return "flash" is seen.

5. **Enter the skin.** Enter the skin with the needle bevel up (for better visualization) and with the ultrasound probe directly over the needle insertion site. To find your needle on the ultrasound image, "bounce," or move the needle a very small amount up and down, without cutting the tissue, and/or swing the needle side to side. As you move the needle tip, you will see it move well on the ultrasound image if you are visualizing the tip. Do not advance the needle until you see the tip of the needle well. Scanning proximally until the needle tip disappears, then scanning distally until the needle tip is again visualized can also assist with ensuring that you are visualizing the tip and not the shaft of the needle.

Table 4.1  **Standard Intravenous Line Types**[*]

| Gauge | Color | Length (mm)[†] | Diameter (mm) | Maximum Flow Rate (mL/min) |
|---|---|---|---|---|
| 14 | Orange | 45 | 2.1 | 240 |
| 16 | Gray | 45 | 1.8 | 180 |
| 18 | Green | 32 | 1.3 | 90 |
| 20 | Pink | 32 | 1.1 | 60 |
| 22 | Blue | 25 | 0.9 | 36 |
| 24 | Yellow | 19 | 0.7 | 20 |

[*] Measurements may vary by manufacturer.
[†] May have several lengths available in each gauge from a given manufacturer.

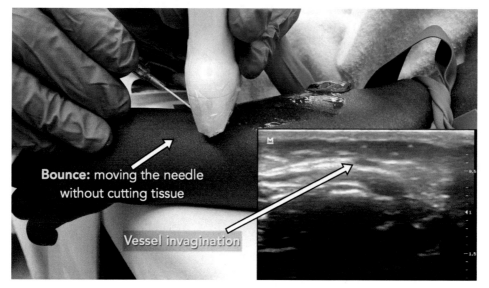

**Figure 4.3** Bouncing the needle on the vein for the purpose of locating the needle tip in relation to the vein.

As you bounce (up and down) on the vein, you will see the needle tip invaginate or indent the vein (Figure 4.3).

> **>> Tip on Technique:** Throughout this procedure, it is very important to put the minimum pressure needed on the ultrasound probe. Pressing down too hard with the ultrasound probe will occlude the vessel and make it very difficult or impossible to cannulate.

---

**Caution!** If the skin is pushed away from the probe or the probe is too close to (on top of) the needle, image dropout will occur (Figure 4.4).

---

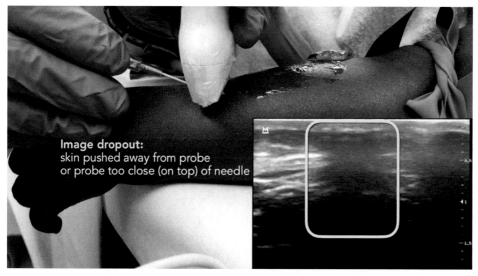

**Figure 4.4** Image dropout.

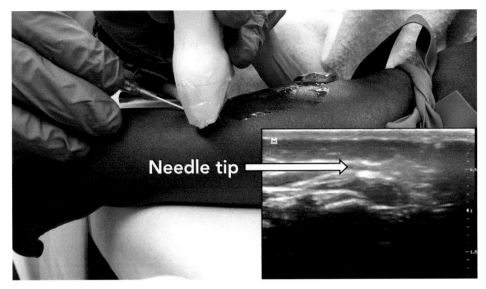

Figure 4.5  Needle tip in vein.

Next, move the needle forward toward the vein while directly visualizing the tip on ultrasound (Figure 4.5). You will see the needle compress the vein on the ultrasound image. Anatomically, the needle is invaginating and dragging the wall of the vessel. As you compress the vein with the needle tip, apply very light pressure until you pop through the vein. After the pop, you will see a target lesion on ultrasound, with the tip of the needle appearing to be in the middle of the lumen of the vein (Figure 4.6).

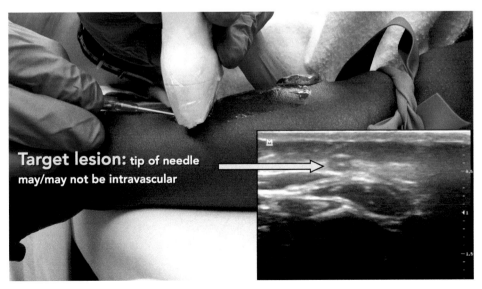

Figure 4.6  Target lesion.

The ultrasound image depicts a "target lesion" ( 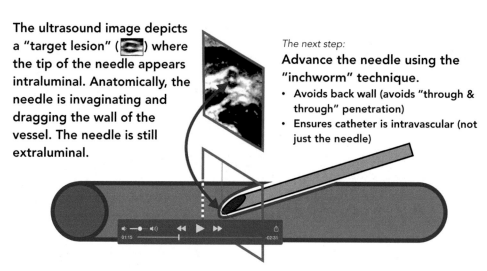 ) where the tip of the needle appears intraluminal. Anatomically, the needle is invaginating and dragging the wall of the vessel. The needle is still extraluminal.

*The next step:*

**Advance the needle using the "inchworm" technique.**

- Avoids back wall (avoids "through & through" penetration)
- Ensures catheter is intravascular (not just the needle)

**Figure 4.7** Although the tip of the needle may be intraluminal, the catheter is likely still extraluminal.

You may or may not see a flash at this point, but you are not done. Although the needle tip may have penetrated the lumen of the vein, the catheter is likely still extraluminal (Figure 4.7).

6. **Advance the needle** under ultrasound guidance by incrementally advancing or "inchworming" the needle forward.

**Incremental Advancement Inchworm Step 1:** Hold the needle steady and nudge the ultrasound probe back and forth (proximally and distally) to identify the tip versus the shaft of the needle (Figure 4.8).

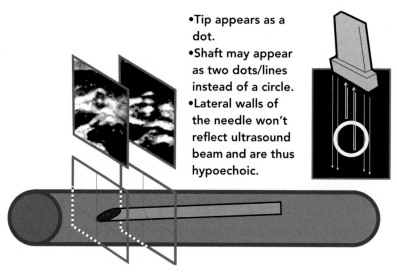

- Tip appears as a dot.
- Shaft may appear as two dots/lines instead of a circle.
- Lateral walls of the needle won't reflect ultrasound beam and are thus hypoechoic.

**Figure 4.8** Viewing the tip versus the shaft of the needle on ultrasound.

## Inchworm, step 1
- hold needle steady
- nudge U/S probe back and forth to identify tip vs. shaft of the needle

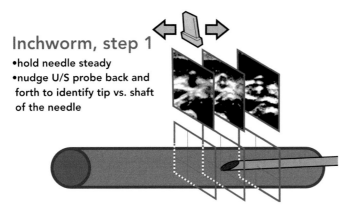

Figure 4.9 Inchworm step 1.

The tip of the needle will appear as a dot. The shaft of the needle may appear as two dots/lines instead of as a circle. The lateral walls of the needle are hypoechoic and therefore will not reflect the ultrasound beam as well as the tip of the needle (Figure 4.9).

**Incremental Advancement Inchworm Step 2:** Nudge the ultrasound probe forward very slightly to the tip of the needle so that you see the needle tip well (keep the tip of the needle within the vessel). Advance the needle 1 to 2 mm. Repeat step 2 until the needle is fully in the vessel (catheter is hubbed at the skin) (Figure 4.10).

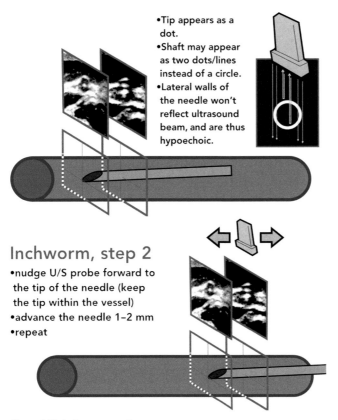

- Tip appears as a dot.
- Shaft may appear as two dots/lines instead of a circle.
- Lateral walls of the needle won't reflect ultrasound beam, and are thus hypoechoic.

## Inchworm, step 2
- nudge U/S probe forward to the tip of the needle (keep the tip within the vessel)
- advance the needle 1–2 mm
- repeat

Figure 4.10 Inchworm step 2.

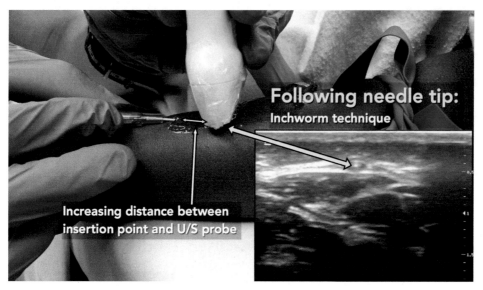

**Figure 4.11** As the inchworm technique proceeds, there will be an increased distance between the insertion point of the needle into the skin and the ultrasound probe.

As the incremental advancement inchworm technique proceeds, there will be an increased distance between the insertion point of the needle into the skin and the ultrasound probe (Figure 4.11).

>> **Tip on Technique:** Proceeding VERY SLOWLY will improve your success rate—the reason this is called the incremental advancement inchworm technique is that the needle is first moved forward the smallest amount possible and very slowly, followed by barely nudging the probe forward very slowly to follow. Using the inchworm technique will help to avoid penetration of the back wall of the vein (i.e., will help avoid going "through and through") and will help to ensure that the catheter is intravascular, not just the tip of the needle.

>> **Tip on Technique:** If you are unsure if the needle/catheter is in the vein, you can turn the probe 90 degrees to obtain a long-axis view and attempt to visualize the entire catheter in the vein. Additionally, while in the long-axis view, you can inject 10 mL of normal saline into the vein under ultrasound guidance, which will allow you to see turbulence within the vein during the injection if the catheter is intravascular. Alternatively, some practitioners use the long-axis view for the entire intravenous line placement.

7. **Remove the tourniquet and secure the intravenous line.** Remove the tourniquet and wipe off the ultrasound gel. Press down on the skin to occlude the vein distal to the catheter tip to decrease the likelihood that blood will spurt out when the needle is removed. Remove the needle. Release distal pressure slightly to ensure that good blood flow from the catheter hub still exists and to fill the catheter hub with blood to avoid entraining air in the intravenous line. Attach the intravenous line to the catheter hub tightly. Cover with a sterile

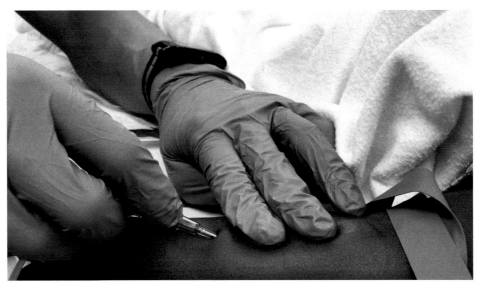

**Figure 4.12** Occluding the vein distally to prevent blood from spurting out of the catheter hub when the needle is removed.

occlusive dressing and tape. Use of a wrap or armboard can assist in decreasing the likelihood that the child will later inadvertently pull out the intravenous line.

---

**Caution!** Avoid circumferential tape and ensure that tapes and wraps are not applied so tightly that circulation is compromised.

---

>> **Tip on Technique:** Avoiding having blood spurt out when the needle is removed can be challenging. The pressure applied to the skin to achieve this must be sufficiently distal that it is past where the tip of the catheter is lying under the skin (Figure 4.12).

## Postoperative Management Considerations

Before the patient is draped, ensure that all connections are tight and that the intravenous line is adequately secured. The intravenous line should be checked regularly for signs of infiltration, phlebitis, or erythema at the site. At the time of removal, pressure should be held for an adequate period of time to ensure hemostasis.

## Acknowledgment

The author would like to thank Michael Woo, MD, for his extensive and generous contributions to the content of this chapter as well as for creating the photos for this chapter.

## Further Reading

Joing S, Strote S, Caroon L, Wall C, et al. Videos in clinical medicine: Ultrasound-guided peripheral i.v. placement. *N Engl J Med.* 2012;366(25):e38.

# References

1. Vinograd AM, Zorc JJ, Dean AJ, et al. First-attempt success, longevity, and complication rates of ultrasound-guided peripheral intravenous catheters in children. *Pediatr Emerg Care.* 2018;34(6):376–380.

2. Doniger SJ, Ishimine P, Fox JC, et al. Randomized controlled trial of ultrasound-guided peripheral intravenous catheter placement versus traditional techniques in difficult-access pediatric patients. *Pediatr Emerg Care.* 2009;25(3):154–159.

3. Au AK, Rotte MJ, Grzybowski RJ, et al. Decrease in central venous catheter placement due to use of ultrasound guidance for peripheral intravenous catheters. *Am J Emerg Med* 2012;30(9):1950–1954.

4. Elia F, Ferrari G, Molino P, et al. Standard-length catheters vs long catheters in ultrasound-guided peripheral vein cannulation. *Am J Emerg Med.* 2012;30(5):712–716.

# Chapter 5

# Arterial Line Placement

*Michael R. King, Ramesh Kodavatiganti, and Hubert A. Benzon*

# ARTERIAL LINE PLACEMENT FUNDAMENTALS

## Introduction

Arterial line placement involves inserting a catheter into a peripheral artery, most commonly the radial or femoral artery. Recent research has also demonstrated the feasibility and ease of cannulation of the posterior tibial artery with the ultrasound technique,[1] although larger studies are needed to assess complication rates. Cannulation of the ulnar, brachial, axillary, dorsalis pedis, and umbilical arteries has also been described. Although the techniques described in this chapter focus on the radial, femoral, and posterior tibial approaches, many of the general principles apply to the other arteries as well.

## Clinical Applications

Arterial lines provide beat-to-beat blood pressure monitoring as well as a readily available means of obtaining blood samples to check arterial blood gas measurements and other labs.

!! **Potential Complications.** Potential complications of an arterial line include hematoma formation, arterial laceration, pseudoaneurysm formation, distal limb ischemia, accidental injection of intravenous medications, and line disconnection leading to hemorrhage. Further data are needed for the pediatric population, but in adults the rate of serious complications from an arterial line requiring a vascular or neurologic consult has been reported at 3.4/10,000.[2]

## Contraindications

While no absolute contraindications exist, many anesthesiologists avoid end-arteries, such as the brachial or dorsalis pedis artery, as sites of cannulation. Avoid extremities at risk of ischemia or with infection or limb compromise.

## Critical Anatomy

The radial artery can be found on the radial aspect of the ventral wrist, and the femoral artery can be found just distal to the inguinal ligament in the medial thigh. Both pulses can be palpated at the skin in a normotensive patient. The radial artery is relatively isolated from major vessels (although typically two small veins run laterally on either side of the radial artery). The femoral artery runs near the femoral nerve and vein. The posterior tibial artery can be palpated behind the medial malleolus. It runs near the tibial nerve and multiple tendons.

| WARNING!! | Avoid attempting cannulation of the ulnar artery if the radial artery has already been attempted and, vice versa, avoid attempting cannulation of the radial artery if the ulnar artery has already been attempted. Many practitioners recommend performing a modified Allen test to assess whether a dual blood supply exists before cannulating either the radial or the ulnar artery. Flow can additionally be assessed by ultrasound or Doppler. |
|---|---|

## Setup

### Equipment
#### For placement:
- Sterile prep and gloves
- Catheter. Specialized arterial catheters are available that include a built-in retractable wire, but these are typically designed for adults. A 24-gauge intravenous catheter is often used for infants, and a 22-gauge catheter is often used for children.

- Guidewire
- Suture and/or liquid adhesive if desired for securing the line
- Sterile dressing

**For connection to the catheter:**
- Pressure tubing and a transducer

# PALPATION TECHNIQUE

## Introduction

See the Arterial Line Placement Fundamentals section for clinical applications, contraindications, critical anatomy, and setup information.

## Step-by-Step

1. **Prepare before the procedure.** Have all the equipment you may need available and nearby when you perform the procedure; it can be difficult to obtain additional supplies when you are in the middle of a procedure. Have multiple catheters and sizes available in case a second attempt is needed.

   >> **Tip on Technique:** Before starting, loosen the catheter from the needle by advancing the catheter slightly off of the needle and then returning the catheter to its original position. This is done so that the catheter will advance easily after blood return "flash" is seen.

2. **Position the patient and prepare the skin.** The radial and femoral arteries will have the straightest course in a fully extended extremity, while the posterior tibial artery will be straightest with the foot in dorsiflexion. Full extension can be achieved for the radial artery with a roll under the wrist and tape applied to abduct the thumb. Take care, however, to avoid overextending the wrist or thumb, which can result in a decreased pulse and a decreased chance of success.

   >> **Tip on Technique:** As you extend the wrist, palpate the artery, and position the wrist at the point of extension with the strongest pulse. Similarly, palpate the artery again as you extend the thumb, and tape the thumb at the point of extension with the strongest pulse.

   The femoral artery can be optimally positioned by abducting the hip. Apply chlorhexidine to sterilize the skin at the insertion site. The posterior tibial artery will be easiest to cannulate with the hip in abduction as well so that the medial malleolus faces up.

   >> **Tip on Technique:** Positioning is key! Maintaining an extended, stable, flat extremity ensures a straighter arterial path as well as a flat surface for palpation or ultrasound placement.

3. **Locate the artery.** Locate the artery by palpating the pulse at the wrist. The course of the artery can be identified by using two fingers placed roughly 1 cm apart along the artery, or by placing the index finger lengthwise down the forearm—the pulse should be felt evenly under the entire finger if the artery is being accurately traced (Figure 5.1).

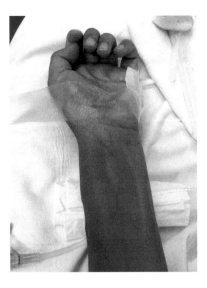

Figure 5.1 Extended wrist.

*Pearl:* Most often, the radial artery is located midway between the lateral edge of the wrist and the lateral-most flexor tendon, and in most patients, the radial artery will course slightly medially as it travels distal to proximal.

>> **Tip on Technique:** Rolling your fingers lightly over the artery can help to locate it and to determine the direction it courses as it goes from lateral to medial. In children and smaller teenagers, you can often feel the outline of the artery using this technique. This can be particularly helpful if the pulse is felt diffusely.

>> **Tip on Technique:** Doppler can be used to determine the point of maximal pulsation. After the location of the artery is determined, press down with the Doppler probe gently to create a slight indentation that will mark the location that you have found.

4. **Insert the needle.** With a finger very lightly on the pulse, insert the needle proximally at a 30- to 45-degree angle into the skin where you feel the location of the artery (Figure 5.2).

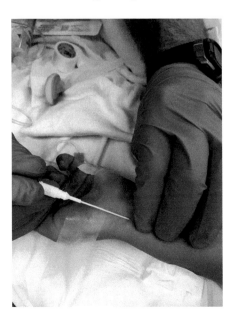

Figure 5.2 Finger on the pulse with an arterial catheter being inserted over the radial artery.

Aim the needle in the direction that you have determined the artery courses as it tracks distally on the arm (will usually be slightly medial).

>> **Tip on technique:** Immediately before entering the skin, some clinicians find it useful to "pull back" on the skin distally with the fifth finger of the hand holding the needle in order to fix the vessel in place.

>> **Tip on Technique:** Go very slowly, advancing a millimeter at a time, and pause for several heartbeats after each advancement—too often, beginners move the needle in and out too quickly, passing by or through the artery with each pass, and thus "shred" the artery with an aggressive technique.

5. **Thread the catheter.** After a flash of blood is seen in the catheter, the clinician should drop the angle and advance slightly, then thread the catheter into the artery (Figure 5.3). If the catheter cannot be threaded off, advancing the needle through the artery and proceeding with a guidewire technique can be useful. To use a guidewire, remove the needle from the catheter and next withdraw the catheter slowly until blood is seen to pulse out, then advance the guidewire though the catheter. Some types of 20- and 22-gauge arterial catheters—such as the one in Figure 5.3—have a built-in wire that can be advanced to ease threading. A specialized small-gauge guidewire is required to fit through 24-gauge catheters.

>> **Tip on Technique:** Alternatively, some clinicians choose to always use a guidewire. To do this, after obtaining pulsatile flow, advance the guidewire beyond the end of the catheter so that it may guide the full insertion of the catheter.

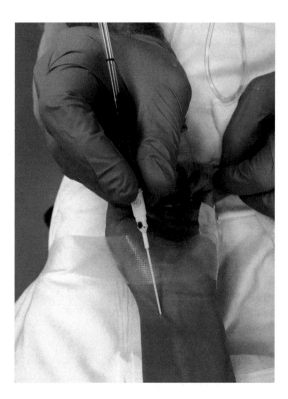

**Figure 5.3** Catheter with "flash" of blood and wire advanced.

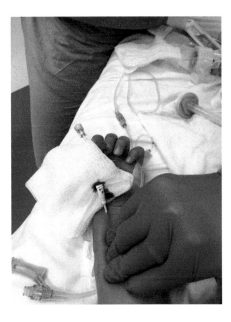

Figure 5.4 Catheter hubbed at the skin.

6. **Advance the catheter.** Advance the catheter (over a wire if needed) until hubbed at the skin. Pressure is held proximally to the catheter to avoid blood loss while the needle or wire is removed and the transduction tubing is attached (Figure 5.4).

   >> **Tip on Technique:** Alternatively, some clinicians choose to start with a through-and-through technique. For this technique, advance the needle through the artery, remove the needle from the angiocatheter, and pull the angiocatheter back until blood is seen to pulse out (Figure 5.5) before advancing the guidewire (Figure 5.6). A through-and-through

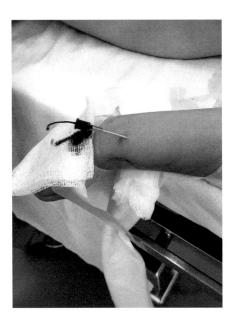

Figure 5.5 Intra-arterial catheter.

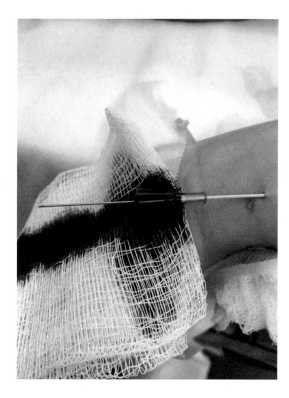

**Figure 5.6** Catheter with guidewire advanced.

technique may increase the likelihood that the catheter has been advanced far enough that both the needle and the cannula will be intra-arterial, and this technique may be useful in patients with very small arteries, such as neonates.

**‼ Potential Complications:** Hematoma formation can result from the through-and-through technique because this technique creates a second puncture in the back of the artery.

## Postoperative Management Considerations

Ensure that the arterial cannulation site, tubing, and any ports of entry are well labeled (e.g. with red tape) to ensure that the arterial line is not mistaken for a venous line. The arterial line should be covered in a sterile fashion after placement and maintained with clean dressings. At the time of removal, pressure should be held until hemostasis is observed. Next, the puncture site should be covered with a sterile occlusive dressing to promote wound healing and prevent infection. Pressure may need to be held for a prolonged period of time in patients who are anticoagulated or coagulopathic.

## ULTRASOUND GUIDED ARTERIAL LINE PLACEMENT

### Introduction

Readers should review the earlier Arterial Line Placement Fundamentals section for clinical applications, contraindications, critical anatomy, and basic setup and equipment information for this procedure.

# Setup

### Additional Equipment

- Sterile ultrasound gel
- Ultrasound machine with a small, high-frequency linear array probe, ideally with a frequency of 7.5 to 10 MHz. A particularly good option in infants and small children is the "hockey-stick" probe, which is small enough to fit on a neonatal wrist and has an angled handle to allow the probe to be gripped away from the field.
- Sterile occlusive dressing or cover for the ultrasound probe

# Step-by-Step

1. **Prepare before the procedure.** Have all equipment you may need available and nearby when you perform the procedure; it can be difficult to obtain additional supplies when you are in the middle of a procedure. Have multiple catheters and sizes available in case a different catheter or second attempt is needed.

    >> **Tip on Technique:** Before starting, loosen the catheter from the needle by advancing the catheter slightly off of the needle and then returning the catheter to its original position. This is done so that the catheter will advance easily after blood return "flash" is seen.

2. **Position the patient and sterilize the skin.** The radial and femoral arteries will have the straightest course in a fully extended extremity. Take care, however, to avoid overextending the wrist or thumb, which can result in a decreased pulse and a decreased chance of success. The femoral artery can be optimally positioned by abducting the hip. Apply chlorhexidine to sterilize the skin at the insertion site.

    >> **Tip on Technique:** Positioning is key! Maintaining an extended, stable, flat extremity ensures a straighter path of the artery as well as a flat surface for palpation or ultrasound guided placement.

3. **Locate the artery.** Place sterile ultrasound gel on the wrist and place the ultrasound probe (covered with a sterile occlusive dressing or cover) on the site. Identify the artery and position it in the middle of the probe/screen. The probe should be aligned on an axis so that the artery remains in the center of the screen when the probe is moved proximally or distally (Figure 5.7A and B).

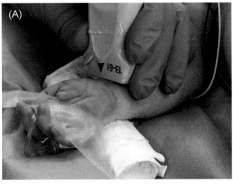 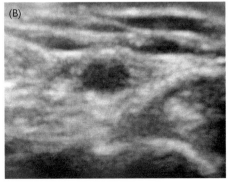

Figure 5.7 (**A**) Wrist positioned in extension with ultrasound in place. (**B**) Ultrasound image of the artery in the middle of the screen.

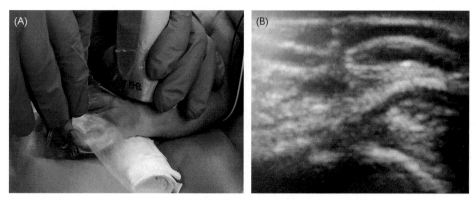

Figure 5.8 (**A**) Needle being inserted into the skin over the artery, distal to the probe at a 30-degree angle. (**B**) An ultrasound image of the needle over the artery.

4. **Insert the needle and locate it on the ultrasound.** Insert the catheter directly in the center of the probe over the artery. Ensure that the catheter is inserted in the direction that the artery has been mapped. Advance the needle toward the probe until the hyperechoic needle can be visualized on the screen (Figure 5.8A and B).

   >> **Tip on Technique:** An alternate technique for ultrasound guided arterial line placement in larger children and teenagers is to use an in-plane view. After placing the artery in the middle of the probe in the out-of-plane view, the probe is rotated 90 degrees to obtain an image of the artery in the in-plane/long-axis view. The needle is inserted in the middle of the probe and visualized on the ultrasound image (Figure 5.9).

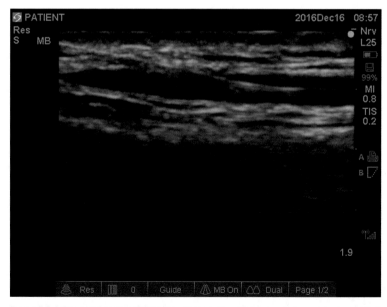

Figure 5.9 Ultrasound image of the artery in long view. The artery in long-axis view with the needle at 45 degrees approaching it.

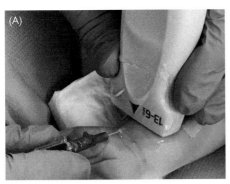
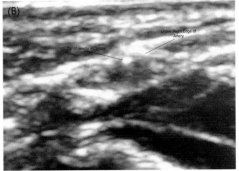

Figure 5.10 (**A**) Flash of blood in the catheter. (**B**) An ultrasound image of the "target sign" of the needle tip in the lumen of the artery.

5. **Advance the needle with ultrasound guidance.** Progressively advance the needle into the artery with ultrasound guidance (Figure 5.10A). Each time the needle is moved forward slightly, the ultrasound should then be moved forward slightly to keep the very tip of the needle visible on the screen (Figure 5.10B). When the needle tip is visualized in the lumen of the artery, blood should be visible in the angiocatheter.

   >> **Tip on Technique:** Going VERY SLOWLY will improve your success rate. We recommend using the incremental advancement or "inchworm" technique in which the tip of the needle is visualized from first puncture until the catheter is fully inserted in the artery. During the incremental advancement technique, the catheter is first advanced forward the smallest amount possible, followed by barely moving the probe forward very slowly to follow. For more details and a video on the incremental advancement technique, which is also used for venous cannulation, see Chapter 4. Compared with venous cannulation, for arterial cannulation, *slightly* more pressure on the angiocatheter may be needed to puncture the artery.

6. **Advance the catheter using ultrasound guidance.** After the needle is in the artery, continue to advance the needle and ultrasound incrementally, visualizing the needle tip during the entire advancement. Continue until the entire catheter has been threaded into the artery under ultrasound visualization (Figure 5.11).

## Postoperative Management Considerations

Ensure that the arterial cannulation site, tubing, and any ports of entry are well labeled (e.g. with red tape) to ensure that the arterial line is not mistaken for a venous line. The arterial line should be covered in a sterile fashion after placement and maintained with clean dressings. At the time of removal, pressure should be held until hemostasis is observed. Next, the puncture site should be covered with a sterile occlusive dressing to promote wound healing and prevent infection. Pressure may need to be held for a prolonged period of time in patients who are anticoagulated or coagulopathic.

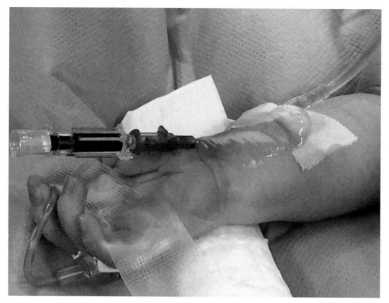

**Figure 5.11** An image of the catheter hubbed with the needle still in place. The back of the catheter has filled with blood.

# CUTDOWN TECHNIQUE

## Introduction

The cutdown technique is a surgical procedure for placing an arterial line. The earlier Arterial Line Placement Fundamentals section provides some information about clinical applications, contraindications, and critical anatomy for arterial lines in general. However, the cutdown technique is a surgical procedure and should only be performed by those with extensive experience in this technique. Typically, it is only performed in cases in which an arterial line is critical for the patient and cannot be placed by conventional means.

## Set-up

### Additional Equipment

- Full surgical sterility, including mask, gown, gloves, sterile prep, sterile drape
- A surgical blade for skin incision
- A surgical probe
- A hemostat
- Ideally, surgical loops for vision

## Step-by-Step

1. **Prepare before the procedure.** The cutdown technique requires a sterile instrument tray. The following items should be included: a blade for incision, probe and hemostat for

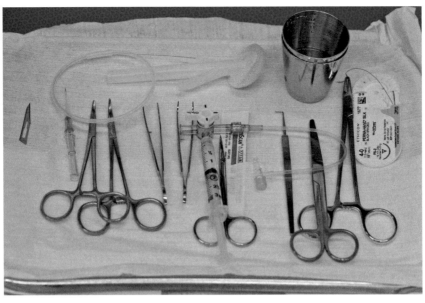

Figure 5.12 Tray with instruments for cutdown technique.

dissection, catheters for cannulation, flush syringe and tubing for connection, and instruments for suturing the arterial line (Figure 5.12).

> **WARNING!!**   If an artery was used for a cutdown arterial line previously, it is advisable to choose a different site because some studies have suggested higher rates of vascular complications with a repeat technique.

2. **Position the patient and prepare the skin.** Extend the wrist, secure it with tape, and prepare the skin in a sterile fashion (Figure 5.13).

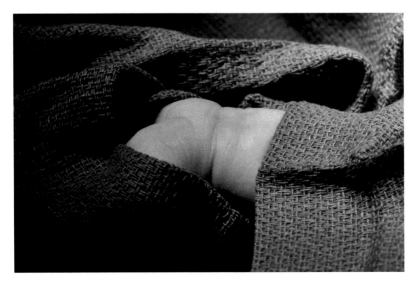

Figure 5.13 Image of an extended wrist covered in sterile blue towels.

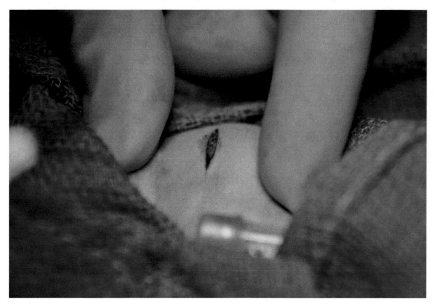

**Figure 5.14** Incised wrist spread by gloved fingers.

3. **Make the incision.** Using a surgical blade, make a 0.5-cm incision centered over the desired artery (Figure 5.14).

---

**WARNING!!**     Although hemorrhage from a failed conventional cannulation is often tamponaded by the skin over the artery, this is not the case in the surgical cutdown technique because the artery will be open to air and can lead to exsanguination unless ligated or packed.

---

4. **Dissect the subcutaneous tissue and expose the artery.** Use a hemostat and probe to separate the tissues within the wrist while looking for linear structures that may be arterial. After dissecting the wrist, use a probe to pull potential arterial structures out of the cavity. The wrist contains veins, nerves, and tendons that appear similar to the artery. Some properties that help to distinguish the artery are vasa vasorum (small vessels in the wall of the artery that are not present in veins) as well as vessel blanching when tension is applied by the probe that resolves when the tension is released (Figure 5.15).

5. **Cannulate the artery.** When the artery is identified, use a probe to hold it steady and under tension while advancing a catheter into the lumen. This is the most critical step because improperly advancing the catheter during arterial dissection can result in uncontrolled hemorrhage or vascular laceration (Figure 5.16).

---

**Caution!**     Blood should continue to be observed pulsing out of the end of the catheter at all stages of needle advancement. If blood is not flowing when the catheter is advanced, the needle is likely in the wall of the artery and will not enter the lumen.

---

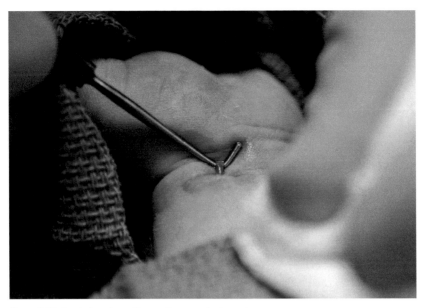

Figure 5.15 Surgical probe pulling up the artery in the wrist.

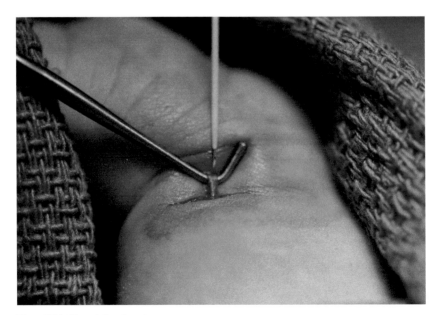

Figure 5.16 Cannulating the artery.

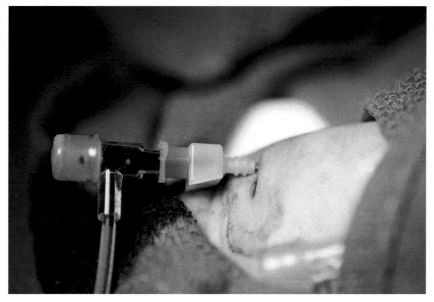

**Figure 5.17** An arterial catheter connected to pressure tubing.

6. **Change the catheter then connect the line.** Once the catheter has been placed, use the Seldinger technique to replace it with a stiffer arterial catheter that is more suitable for arterial use. Connect the catheter to pressure tubing (Figure 5.17).

7. **Secure the cannula.** Use a suture to close the skin incision (at least one stitch on either side of the arterial catheter). Suture the cannula in place. Dress the site in a sterile fashion (Figure 5.18).

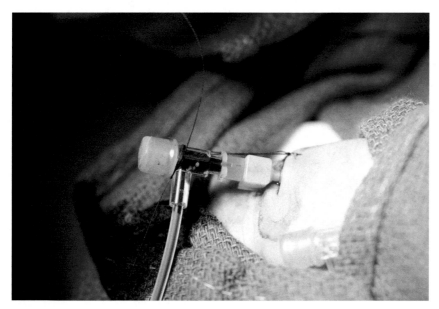

**Figure 5.18** The arterial line and tubing sutured securely.

## Postoperative Management Considerations

Ensure that the arterial cannulation site, tubing, and any ports of entry are well labeled (e.g. with red tape) to ensure that the arterial line is not mistaken for a venous line. The arterial line should be covered with a sterile dressing. A cutdown arterial line should be removed by someone familiar with how the insertion procedure and securing of the line were accomplished. At the time of removal, pressure should be held until hemostasis is observed, and then the site should be covered with a sterile occlusive dressing to promote wound healing and prevent infection. Pressure may need to be held for a prolonged period of time in patients who are anticoagulated or coagulopathic, and on rare occasion, a vascular surgeon may be needed to repair the vessel.

## Further Reading

Aouad-Maroun M, Raphael CK, Sayyid SK, et al. Ultrasound-guided arterial cannulation for paediatrics. *Cochrane Database Syst Rev.* 2016;9:cd011364.

Miyasaka K, Edmonds JF, Conn AW. Complications of radial artery lines in the paediatric patient. *Can Anaesth Soc J.* 1976; 23(1):9–14.

Schindler E, Kowald B, Suess H, et al. Catheterization of the radial or brachial artery in neonates and infants. *Paediatr Anaesth.* 2005; 15(8):677–682.

## References

1. Kim EH, Lee JH, Song IK, Kim JT, Lee WJ, Kim HS. Posterior tibial artery as an alternative to the radial artery for arterial cannulation site in small children: a randomized controlled study. *Anesthesiology.* 2017;127(3):423–431.
2. Nuttall G, Burckhardt J, Hadley A, et al. Surgical and patient risk factors for severe arterial line complications in adults. *Anesthesiology.* 2016;124(3):590–597.

5. Arterial Line Placement

# Chapter 6

# Central Venous Catheter Placement Using the Seldinger Technique

*Kirk Lalwani and Philip W. Yun*

# CENTRAL VENOUS ACCESS FUNDAMENTALS

## Introduction

Central venous access is commonly achieved through the internal jugular, subclavian, or femoral vein. Each site presents its own risks and challenges. Among the considerations for determining the optimal site of insertion for each patient are age, duration of intended use, operator expertise, and the need for sedation. In children, central lines are often placed under general anesthesia or heavy sedation to decrease the risk for patient movement.

## Clinical Applications

Central venous access may be indicated for monitoring central venous pressure, administration of hyperosmolar or vasoactive medications, hemodialysis, or rapid infusion of fluids.

## Contraindications

Each patient should be considered individually. Risks versus benefits should be weighed in the coagulopathic patient. The femoral site may be preferred if a central line is required in a coagulopathic patient because the femoral site is more easily compressed. Consider administration of fresh frozen plasma before line placement in the coagulopathic patient.

---

**WARNING!!**  To decrease the likelihood of air embolus, place the patient in the Trendelenburg position before starting central line placement and maintain this position during the procedure. Also use the Trendelenburg position during central line removal.

---

## Types of Central Lines

When placing a central line, commonly used veins are the internal jugular, subclavian, and femoral. Use of the external jugular vein is less common.

### Internal Jugular

Positioning is key when placing an internal jugular central venous line; a shoulder roll is helpful to pull back the shoulders and maximally expose the neck. The patient's head should be turned to the contralateral side. Trendelenburg positioning helps to engorge the internal jugular vein for better visualization and may decrease the risk for air embolus. When placing a central line in the internal jugular vein, real-time ultrasound is recommended and has become the standard of care if available.[1] With the patient supine and in the Trendelenburg position, the needle is inserted under ultrasound guidance and directed toward the patient's ipsilateral nipple (Figure 6.1). Figure 6.2 shows an internal jugular line in situ after placement of the line and sterile dressing.

---

**Caution!**  The carotid artery lies medial to the internal jugular vein. Use ultrasound guidance to locate the best access point for the internal jugular vein and avoid inadvertent arterial puncture.

---

**!! Potential Complications:** Potential complications include hematoma, arterial puncture/cannulation, pneumothorax, infection, and thrombus formation.

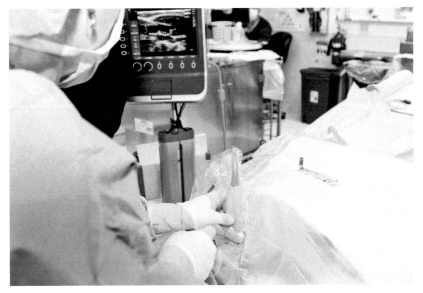

**Figure 6.1** Internal jugular central venous line being inserted under ultrasound guidance.

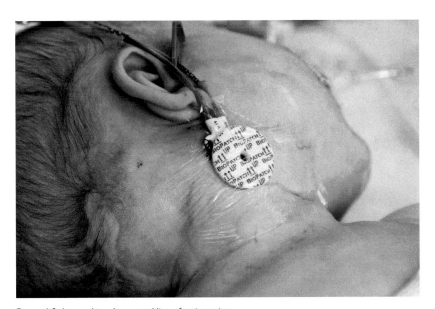

**Figure 6.2** Internal jugular central line after insertion.

## Subclavian

With the patient supine and in the Trendelenburg position, the needle is inserted inferior to the lateral third of the clavicle and directed toward the sternal notch (Figure 6.3). The left side is preferred if there are no contraindications because on the right side, the subclavian-jugular venous junction overlies the subclavian artery (Figure 6.4).[2] With the initial attempt, advance the needle at a shallow angle parallel to the chest wall to minimize the risk for arterial puncture or

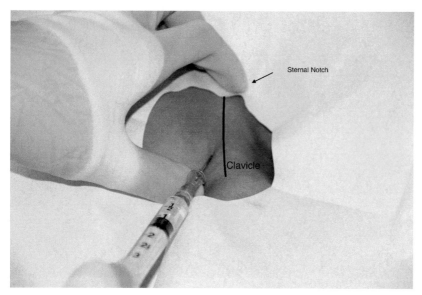

**Figure 6.3** Subclavian central venous line placement.

pneumothorax. Elevation of the chest can be achieved with a towel between the back of the shoulders. Trendelenburg positioning helps engorge the subclavian vein to create a larger target for cannulation. Figure 6.4 shows a subclavian line in situ after placement of the central line and sterile dressing.

**‼ Potential Complications:** Attempted placement of a subclavian central line may result in serious complications, including pneumothorax and hemothorax, hematoma, arterial

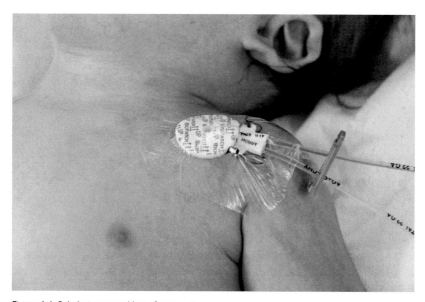

**Figure 6.4** Subclavian central line after insertion.

puncture/cannulation, infection, and thrombus formation. Thoracic duct injury can also occur with left-sided placement.

### Femoral

When placing a central line in the femoral vein, the patient is placed supine with the legs in slight external rotation. Use the mnemonic "NAVEL" for nerve, artery, vein, empty space, and lymphatics from lateral to medial to remember the anatomy of the femoral triangle. Continuous ultrasound during needle placement can be used and is associated with a higher first-attempt success rate and fewer attempts overall.[3] If an ultrasound is not available, the artery is palpated and the vein is approached just medial to the artery. Direct the needle toward the umbilicus.

**!! Potential Complications:** Potential complications include hematoma, arterial puncture/cannulation, infection, and thrombus formation.

### External Jugular

When a central line is to be placed in the external jugular vein, the patient should be positioned supine and in the Trendelenburg position. The Trendelenburg position and distal manual compression may improve visibility by increasing venous distension.

**!! Potential Complications:** Potential complications include hematoma, infection, thrombus formation, and difficulty with placement.

## Setup

### Equipment

- Sterile gloves/gowns/drapes
- Face mask
- Central line kit (needle, syringe, wire, dilator, scalpel, age-appropriate catheter) (Figure 6.5)

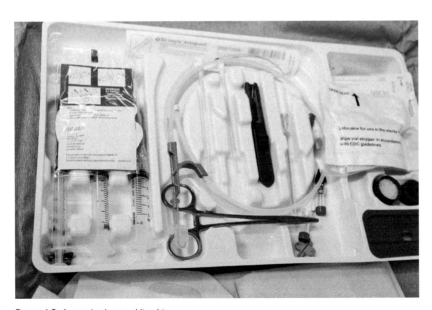

**Figure 6.5** A standard central line kit.

- Suture/dressing
- If desired, an ultrasound machine and sterile cover for the ultrasound probe

The catheter gauge and length are chosen based on the patient's age and size as well as the clinical situation. A guide to commonly used sizes is in Table 6.1. A general rule of thumb for initial length of insertion of the catheter is:

**Table 6.1 Commonly Used Central Line Sizes by Age**

| Age (yr) | Weight (kg) | Gauge | French |
|----------|-------------|-------|--------|
| Neonate | <4 | 24 | 3.0 |
| <1 | 5–10 | 22 | 3.0 |
| 1–2 | 10–12 | 20 or 22 | 3.0–3.5 |
| 3–5 | 12–20 | 18 or 20 | 4.0–4.5 |
| 6–10 | 20–30 | 18 or 20 | 4.5 or higher |
| >10 | >30 | 16, 18, or 20 | 5.0–8.0 |

**For patients ≤100 cm in height:**
   Correct length of insertion (cm) = (height in cm/10) − 1
**For patients >100 cm in height:**
   Correct length of insertion (cm) = (height in cm/10) − 2

One study predicted that using these formulae, the central venous catheter would be above the right atrium in 97% of internal jugular or subclavian catheter insertions.[4]

>> **Tip on Technique:** Before beginning the procedure, flush all of the ports of the central venous catheter with saline and clamp the ports to avoid loss of saline and decrease the likelihood of entraining air into the patient when the line is placed.

## THE SELDINGER TECHNIQUE

## Step-by-Step

1. **Prepare for the procedure, position the patient appropriately, and sterilize the patient's skin** (see the previous section on Central Venous Access Fundamentals). Ensure availability of all necessary equipment and supplies and the proper positioning of the patient. Prepare the skin with aseptic solution and use maximum sterile barrier precautions throughout.[5] For the internal/external jugular and subclavian approaches, place the patient in a slightly head-down position to decrease the likelihood of air entrainment through the vein during the procedure.

   >> **Tip on Technique:** Before puncturing the vein, ensure that the syringe can be easily removed from the needle and that the catheter can be slid from the needle with ease.

2. **Puncture the vein.** Using landmark or ultrasound guidance (Figure 6.6), advance the needle with the syringe attached into the vein while simultaneously aspirating with the syringe. Once blood is freely aspirated through the syringe, stabilize the needle with your left hand against

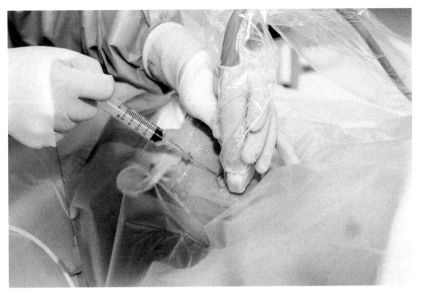

**Figure 6.6** Using continuous ultrasound for venipuncture of the internal jugular vein.

the patient's body to ensure that the needle does not move. Particularly in neonates and infants, small movements can accidentally dislodge the needle from the vein.

>> **Tip on Technique:** In the infant, vessels are easily compressible and of small caliber. For this reason, when placing a central line in an infant, it may be necessary, after the initial puncture, to withdraw slowly with continuous syringe aspiration to access the vein.

>> **Tip on Technique:** Ensure free flow of blood or easy aspiration with a syringe before inserting the guidewire.

---

**WARNING!!**  After removing the needle and before placing the wire, and on any occasion that the central vein could entrain air, occlude the catheter with your sterile finger.

---

>> **Tip on Technique:** Before starting central line placement, prepare the wire for insertion and place within reach to minimize the chance of inadvertently moving the needle out of the vein while reaching for the wire. In pediatric patients, even a few millimeters of motion can displace the needle from the vein.

3. **Advance the wire through the needle and confirm venous placement.** Remove the syringe and gently advance the wire through the needle. Confirm that the wire is positioned in the vein with the following methods: (1) Visualize the wire in the vein on ultrasound; (2) advance an angiocatheter over the wire, then remove the wire and transduce the angiocatheter to confirm the central venous waveform and pressure. Then, readvance the wire over the angiocatheter. The wire should easily advance through the needle (Figure 6.7).

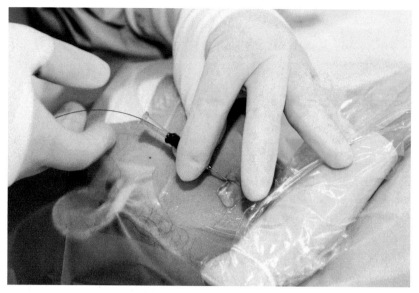

Figure 6.7 The wire should easily advance through the needle.

**WARNING!!**    Withdrawal of the wire through the needle may shear off the end of the wire intravascularly, especially with smaller diameter wires. Do not reuse a damaged wire.

**Caution!**    Advancement of the wire into the heart can elicit ectopic beats. If this occurs, withdraw the wire out of the heart. Ectopic beats also serve as a sign that the wire is going down through the vein into the superior vena cava.

4. **Dilate the vein.** While keeping the wire in place, remove the needle (or angiocatheter). Load the dilator onto the wire. Insert the tip of the scalpel alongside the wire with the sharp side of the blade pointing upward (this allows the cutting motion to be directed superficially to avoid external jugular vein damage). Make a skin nick with the scalpel along the wire just large enough to allow for easy passage of the dilator along the wire and into the patient (Figure 6.8). Insert the dilator into the patient along the wire, then remove the dilator from the wire, taking care to keep control of the wire at all times.

**Caution!**    When placing an internal jugular central venous line, ensure that the skin nick is away from the external jugular vein.

>> **Tip on Technique:** Loading the dilator onto the wire before the skin nick allows for quick advancement of the dilator to minimize bleeding from the incision.

5. **Thread the central venous catheter along the wire.** Thread the catheter over the wire to the desired depth and then remove the wire. Advance the catheter along the wire while maintaining manual control of the wire proximally (Figure 6.9).

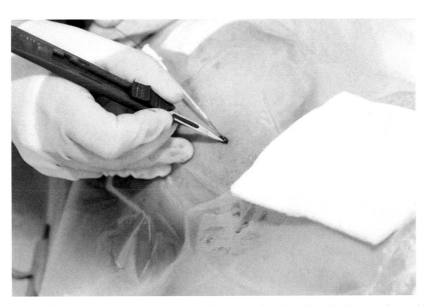

Figure 6.8 Dilator prepared to be inserted into the patient along the wire, with clinician making a skin nick.

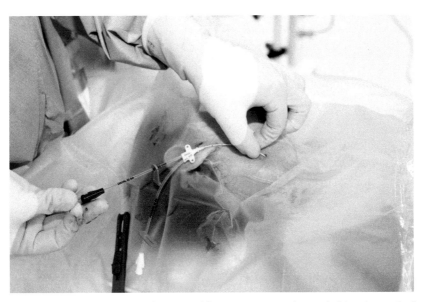

Figure 6.9 Advance the catheter along wire while maintaining manual control of the wire proximally.

6. **Secure the catheter and apply the dressing.** Secure the catheter with a suture or other securing device and apply an occlusive dressing over the insertion site. Aspirate from all lumens and flush each lumen. Clamp each lumen after flushing with saline.

## Postoperative Management Considerations

> **WARNING!!** Place the patient in Trendelenburg position during removal of an upper body central venous catheter to decrease the risk for a potentially fatal air embolism.

Central venous catheters should be removed as soon as possible if they are no longer indicated because a central venous catheter is a site that is at risk for infection.[6]

## Further Reading

Rupp SM, Apfelbaum JL, Blitt C, et al. Practice guidelines for central venous access: a report by the American Society of Anesthesiologists Task Force on Central Venous Access. *Anesthesiology.* 2012;116:539–573.

## References

1. Verghese ST, McGill WA, Patel RI, et al. Comparison of three techniques for internal jugular vein cannulation in infants. *Paediatr Anaesth.* 2000;10:505–511.
2. Tarbiat M, Manafi B, Davoudi M, Totonchi Z. Comparison of the complications between left side and right side subclavian vein catheter placement in patients undergoing coronary artery bypass graft surgery. *J Cardiovasc Thorac Res.* 2014;6(3):147–151.
3. Aouad MT, Kanazi GE, Abdallah FW, et al. Femoral vein cannulation performed by residents: a comparison between ultrasound-guided and landmark technique in infants and children undergoing cardiac surgery. *Anesth Analg.* 2010;111:724–728.
4. Andropoulos DB, Bent ST, Skjonsby B, Stayer SA. The optimal length of insertion of central venous catheters for pediatric patients. *Anesth Analg.* 2001;93(4):883–886.
5. Raad II, Hohn DC, Gilbreath BJ, et al. Prevention of central venous catheter-related infections by using maximal sterile barrier precautions during insertion. *Infect Control Hosp Epidemiol.* 1994;15:231–238.
6. Jonge RC, Polderman KH, Gemke RJ. Central venous catheter use in the pediatric patient: mechanical and infectious complications. *Pediatr Crit Care Med.* 2005;6:329–339.

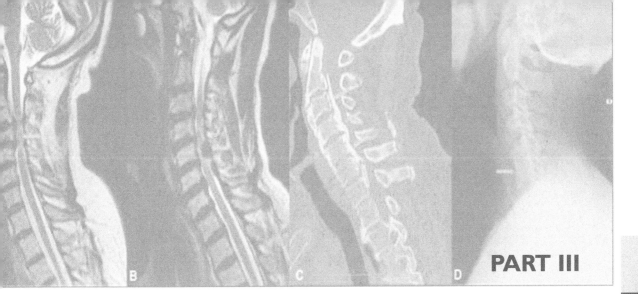

# ULTRASOUND GUIDED PEDIATRIC REGIONAL ANESTHESIA

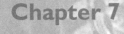

# Chapter 7

# Special Considerations of Regional Anesthesia in Pediatric Patients

*Anna Clebone*

# Introduction

Before 2007, many unanswered questions about best practice for pediatric regional anesthesia existed. These questions included: Is regional anesthesia safe under general anesthesia? Are peripheral nerve catheters safe in the pediatric population? What is a safe dose of local anesthetic in a child? Obviously, it would be very difficult, if not impossible, to gain approval by an institutional review board for a prospective trial to answer these questions.

Luckily, the Pediatric Regional Anesthesia Network was founded in 2007 to help address just such questions. Participating centers (now 21 centers) accrue data on every regional anesthetic procedure performed at that center starting on the day of enrollment. More than 100,000 pediatric regional and neuraxial anesthetics have been logged. In addition to serving as a research repository, the database allows each department to compare its practice with other institutions.

# Regional Anesthesia in Children

### Safety of Regional Anesthesia Under General Anesthesia in Children

In the Pediatric Regional Anesthesia Network (PRAN) database, the safety of regional anesthesia is high: the incidence of transient neurologic deficits after regional anesthesia under general anesthesia is very low (2.4/10,000), and there are no cases of permanent neurologic deficit.[1,2] According to the European Society for Regional Anesthesia (ESRA)/American Society for Regional Anesthesia (ASRA) Guidelines for Pediatric Regional Anesthesia, performing pediatric regional anesthesia under general anesthesia or deep sedation is the standard of care.[3] All safety precautions should be taken, and patients should be carefully monitored and followed.

### Risk for Local Anesthetic Systemic Toxicity Under General Anesthesia in Children

In the PRAN database, local anesthetic systemic toxicity did not occur more often in pediatric patients undergoing regional anesthesia under general anesthesia than in patients undergoing regional anesthesia awake or under sedation, and was overall very rare (2.2/10,000 and 15.2/10,000, respectively).[1,2] However, despite these findings, clinicians should keep in mind that neurologic or cardiac toxicity related to excessive local anesthetic blood concentration is more likely to occur in infants because of low protein binding and decreased intrinsic clearance of local anesthetics in this population. Therefore, heightened vigilance is necessary when administering regional anesthesia under general anesthesia to infants.

### Should a Test Dose Be Used?

A test dose of local anesthetic is commonly used in regional anesthesia to evaluate the possibility of intravascular placement of the block needle or catheter. A test dose should not be considered to be conclusive because signs and symptoms are blunted under general anesthesia or deep sedation and a misplacement of the catheter may be only partly intravascular.[3] To decrease the risk for toxicity, any dose of local anesthetic should be administered slowly, with incremental aspiration every 0.1 to 0.2 mL/kg and with continuous monitoring of and attention paid to the vital signs and electrocardiogram tracing.[3] According to the ESRA/ASRA Guidelines for Pediatric Regional Anesthesia, in the space of time encompassing 30 to 90 seconds immediately following local anesthetic injection, a change in the T wave or heart rate should be considered to be indicative of accidental intravenous injection of local anesthetic,[3] even if blood is not seen during catheter or needle aspiration.

### Safety of Placing an Indwelling Catheter to Anesthetize a Peripheral Nerve

The safety of placing an indwelling catheter to anesthetize a peripheral nerve has also been demonstrated in children, with a complication rate similar to that seen in adults, again using the PRAN database.[4] Although the risk for neurologic injury is low, safety precautions must be taken. Specifically, if during a postoperative continuous regional anesthetic, a motor block occurs that is not anticipated, the infusion should be stopped and an evaluation should be performed because of the concomitant "high index of suspicion for neurologic injury."[3]

## Conclusion

The safety of regional anesthesia in children by expert practitioners is well established. Large database studies show that local anesthetic systemic toxicity and transient neurologic deficits are rare. Practitioners should keep in mind that the centers studied in the PRAN database used all safety precautions and that regional anesthesia was performed by experienced practitioners at these centers. Regional anesthesia should always be performed with all safety precautions taken and by those practitioners with expert training in the technique.

## References

1. Taenzer AH, Walker BJ, Bosenberg AT, et al. Asleep versus awake: does it matter? Pediatric regional block complications by patient state: a report from the Pediatric Regional Anesthesia Network. *Reg Anesth Pain Med.* 2014;39(4):279–283.
2. Walker BJ, Long JB, Sathyamoorthy M, et al. Complications in pediatric regional anesthesia: an analysis of more than 100,000 blocks from the Pediatric Regional Anesthesia Network. *Anesthesiology.* 2018;129(4):721–732.
3. Ivani G, Suresh S, Ecoffey C, et al. The European Society of Regional Anaesthesia and Pain Therapy and the American Society of Regional Anesthesia and Pain Medicine Joint Committee practice advisory on controversial topics in pediatric regional anesthesia. *Reg Anesth Pain Med.* 2015;40(5):526–532.
4. Walker BJ, Long JB, De Oliveira GS, et al. Peripheral nerve catheters in children: an analysis of safety and practice patterns from the pediatric regional anesthesia network (PRAN). *Br J Anaesth.* 2015;115(3):457–462.

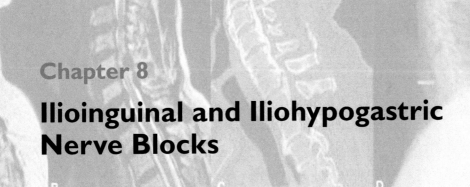

# Chapter 8

# Ilioinguinal and Iliohypogastric Nerve Blocks

*Ann Lawrence and Corey Sheahan*

# Introduction

Ilioinguinal and iliohypogastric nerve blocks are performed by injecting local anesthetic into the facial layer between the internal oblique and transversus abdominis muscles, with the goal of anesthetizing the nerves that originate from the L1 spinal root. This block provides analgesia to a) the skin over the lower abdomen where it joins with the upper pelvis, b) the upper pelvis, and c) along the middle portion of the thigh. Historically, a blind technique was utilized, during which the needle was inserted until a palpable "fascial click" was felt. This approach had an estimated 20 to 30% failure rate as well as a higher risk for iatrogenic small bowel and colonic puncture. An ultrasound guided approach reduces the risk for complications and has been shown to be successful, reducing postoperative analgesia requirements as well as reducing the volume of local anesthetic required.[1] Therefore, an ultrasound guided technique is recommended. An ilioinguinal/iliohypogastric block is a "field block," meaning that the goal is to inject local anesthetic in the plane between the internal oblique and transverse abdominis muscles, which will adequately block the nerve, even when the nerve itself is not visualized.

# Clinical Applications

An ilioinguinal/iliohypogastric block can provide intraoperative and postoperative analgesia for most surgeries in the inguinal area, for example, inguinal hernia repair or orchiopexy.[1] In children, an ilioinguinal/iliohypogastric block is almost always performed under general anesthesia and may be effective in reducing opioid requirements during both the intraoperative and postoperative periods.[2] An ilioinguinal/iliohypogastric block can be as effective as a caudal block, with a lower volume of local anesthetic required.[3]

# Contraindications

Few absolute contraindications to an ilioinguinal/iliohypogastric nerve block exist. Contraindications include infection at the puncture site, true allergy to local anesthetics, anticoagulant therapy, and parental or patient refusal. Nerve blocks in patients with degenerative axonal pathology have long been debated, and limited data exist on the topic. Unless a strong indication exists, in which the benefits outweigh the risks, it is suggested that regional anesthetic procedures be avoided in patients with degenerative axonal pathology.[4] Regional anesthesia in patients with congenital blood disorders such as hemophilia, von Willebrand disease, and specific clotting factor deficiencies remain controversial as well because no randomized controlled trials exist for regional anesthesia in these populations.

# Critical Anatomy

The L1 primary ventral ramus originates from the lumbar plexus. L1 traverses the psoas major where it branches into the ilioinguinal and iliohypogastric nerves, which emerge at the lateral border of the psoas major. These two nerves then travel through the lumbar fascia and follow the plane between the internal oblique and transversus abdominis. The anatomy is relatively unchanged between the pediatric and adult population with the exception that the distance from the anterior-superior iliac spine is estimated to be 5 to 15 mm in children.[5]

# Setup

## Equipment

- 22- to 25-gauge echogenic regional block needle
- Ultrasound machine with linear probe array and sterile probe cover or sterile occlusive dressing to cover the probe

- Sterile ultrasound gel
- Sterile gloves
- Sterile preparation solution
- Sterile towels or other sterile drape

| **WARNING!!** | Alcohol-based skin preparation solutions are a potential fire hazard in the operating room, especially when electrocautery is utilized for the surgical procedure. When using an alcohol-based skin prep, do not allow excess preparation solution to pool around or under the patient. Ensure that the alcohol-based skin preparation solution is completely dry and that any excess is wiped away with towels before preparing the patient for surgery. |
|---|---|

- 20% intralipid readily available

**Drugs, Dosages, Administration**

| **WARNING!!** | It is important to calculate the allowable total local anesthetic dose by weight and to stay below this maximum dose in order to decrease the risk for local anesthetic systemic toxicity. This calculation should include all local anesthetics, including that given by the surgeon, intravenous (IV) local anesthetic given by the anesthesiologist, and EMLA or subcutaneous lidocaine given before starting an IV line. |
|---|---|

The previously recommended dose for ilioinguinal/iliohypogastric nerve blocks was 0.25 mL/kg of 0.25% bupivacaine or ropivacaine; however, if the nerves are sufficiently surrounded, local anesthetic doses as low as 0.075 mL/kg will still provide an effective block.[6]

Before the start of the case, gather all of the necessary equipment. Based on the patient's body weight, calculate an appropriate dose of local anesthetic and adjuvant (if desired).

>> **Tip on Technique:** It may be useful to gather all supplies on a mobile flat surface, such as a mayo stand, to utilize for equipment setup during the procedure.

| **Caution!** | Double-check your patient's allergies before collection of medications and antiseptic solutions. |
|---|---|

## Step-by-Step

1. **Prepare before the procedure.** Place standard American Society of Anesthesiologists monitors on the child and then administer a general anesthetic by intravenous or inhalational techniques. Place the intravenous line, if it is not already in situ, and secure the airway as desired for the surgical procedure. The block itself is performed either before or after the surgical procedure.

*Pearl:* Performing the block before the surgical procedure can assist with surgical analgesia, decreasing the need for opioid dosing during the surgery. Some surgeons, however, have the opinion that the fluid injected near the surgical site interferes with surgical visualization and therefore prefer that the block be performed after the completion of the surgery.

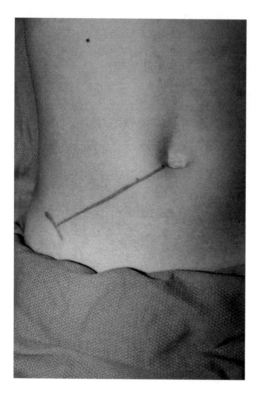

Figure 8.1 The patient's abdomen and pelvis are exposed so that a line from the ipsilateral anterior-superior iliac spine to the umbilicus can be easily visualized.

2. **Position the patient, identify landmarks, and prepare the skin.** For the ilioinguinal/iliohypogastric nerve block, the child should remain supine with the abdominal and inguinal region exposed. The most critical anatomical landmark is the ipsilateral anterior-superior iliac spine. If desired, a marking pen may be used to draw a line from the anterior-superior iliac spine to the umbilicus (Figure 8.1). This line will act as a guide for the trajectory of the ultrasound probe. Using sterile gloves and sterile prep solution, clean a wide circular area of skin on the side on which you are performing the block, from the anterior-superior iliac spine to the umbilicus.

> **WARNING!!**   Chlorhexidine topical solution is not recommended for use in premature infants or infants younger than 2 months because of the risks for irritation or chemical burn and potential systemic absorption.[7]

3. **Place the ultrasound probe.** Carefully place a sterile sheath over the ultrasound probe. Place the ultrasound probe against the anterior-superior iliac spine with the linear probe oriented along the line between the anterior-superior iliac spine and the umbilicus (Figure 8.2).

4. **Visualize the muscles and nerves.** From superficial to deep, the layers that will be visualized on ultrasound are fat (may be minimal in children), external oblique, internal oblique, transverse abdominis, and the peritoneal cavity. The internal oblique and transverse abdominis muscles should be fairly easy to view; however, in about half of pediatric patients, the external oblique cannot be visualized.[2] Although it is not necessary to visualize the nerve (i.e., because it is a field block), the ilioinguinal nerve typically lies between the internal oblique and transverse abdominis muscles and should appear as a distinct hypoechoic structure (Figure 8.3). The iliohypogastric nerve travels adjacent and medial to the ilioinguinal nerve.[8]

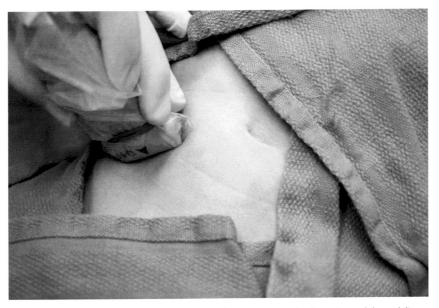

Figure 8.2 An ultrasound probe is placed between the anterior-superior iliac spine and the umbilicus.

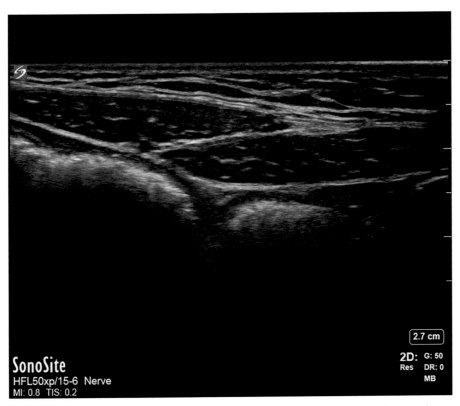

Figure 8.3 The ilioinguinal and iliohypogastric nerves are the hypoechoic structure that lies between the internal oblique and transverse abdominis muscles.

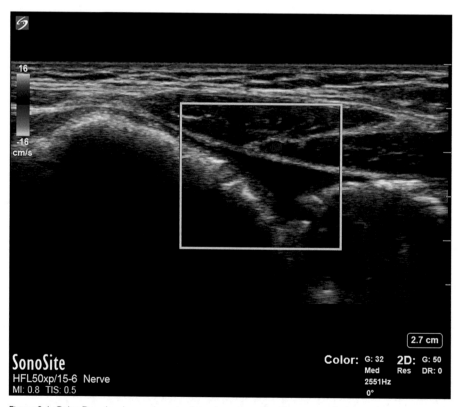

>> **Tip on Technique**: If these three muscle layers are difficult to visualize, the following technique can be used: Scan nearby (up, down, lateral, or medial) until the three distinct muscle layers are visualized. Next, scan back to the ilioinguinal area, following the plane between the internal oblique and transverse abdominis layers as you scan. Another technique is to visualize the peritoneum (often you will see peristalsis on ultrasound), then look at the layers above the peritoneum (first layer above is the transverse abdominis, second layer above is the internal oblique, and the ilioinguinal and iliohypogastric nerves lie between these two layers).

>> **Tip on Technique**: Another technique for locating the plane between the internal oblique and the transverse abdominis muscles is to use color Doppler. Color Doppler may be used to locate a branch of the deep circumflex iliac artery, which lies in the same anatomical plane as the ilioinguinal and iliohypogastric nerves (Figure 8.4). The location of the deep circumflex iliac artery may be used to verify the proper anatomical plane.[8]

5. **Place the needle under ultrasound guidance.** Once an optimal ultrasound image is obtained, insert the block needle about 0.5 cm lateral to the transducer. Advance the needle in-plane under direct visualization with the probe toward the target nerve/fascial plane while avoiding vascular structures (Figure 8.5). If the nerve has not been visualized, position the needle

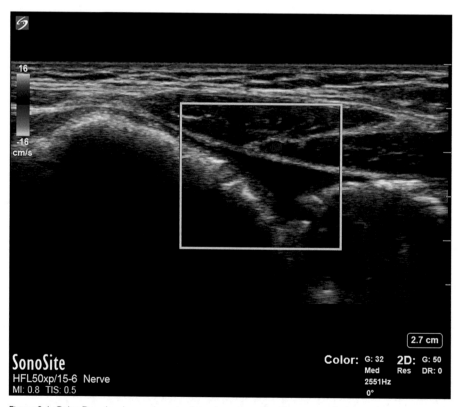

Figure 8.4 Color Doppler shows a branch of the deep circumflex iliac artery, which lies adjacent to the two nerves.

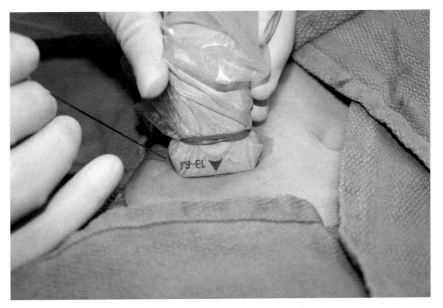

Figure 8.5 Needle approaching the skin in-plane to the ultrasound probe.

tip between the internal oblique and transverse abdominis layers. If the nerve is visualized, position the needle slightly outside the nerve sheath. With the local anesthetic syringe, gently aspirate. If blood is visualized, do not inject the local anesthetic solution. Reposition the needle and repeat the previous steps until aspiration is negative. If aspiration is negative, inject approximately 1 mL of solution and observe for local anesthetic spread on ultrasound (Figure 8.6). Injection of local anesthetic solution into the correct location between the internal oblique and transverse abdominis muscles can be verified by visualizing the peritoneum pushed downward by injection of the solution. Repeat aspiration after every 1 to 2 mL of anesthetic solution delivered.

**WARNING!!** Because of the close proximity of this regional anesthesia location to the abdominal cavity and the intestines, it is possible to cause a colonic or small bowel puncture or potentially a pelvic hematoma, although this is rare.[1] Needle placement and injection of the local anesthetic solution in a plane below where intended may lead to inadvertent femoral nerve block.[2] Intravascular injection of bupivacaine or ropivacaine during the placement of the block may result in local anesthetic toxicity. This may be seen as hypotension, rhythm disturbance, altered consciousness, seizures, or even cardiac arrest. Negative aspiration before each incremental injection of local anesthetic and continuous monitoring are critical to minimize the chance of local anesthetic systemic toxicity.

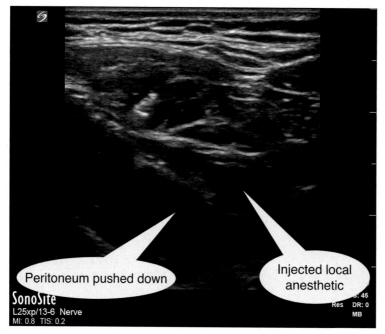

**Figure 8.6** The iliohypogastric and ilioinguinal nerves are seen as the hypoechoic structure floating in a deposit of local anesthetic.

## Postoperative Management Considerations

In patients with a functioning regional anesthetic, opioid requirements may be reduced. Caregivers should be warned to expect the need for analgesia to increase as the block slowly "wears off." The sensation over the area blocked will remain decreased for approximately 4 to 6 hours, similar to a caudal block.[10] Caregivers should be told to carefully place their child in a car seat or seat belt so as to avoid injury to the surgical area. Additionally, a dose of oral pain medication should be considered before the regional anesthetic wears off, depending on the anticipated level of pain from the surgery.

## References

1. Willschke H, Marhofer P, Bösenberg A, et al. Ultrasonography for ilioinguinal/iliohypogastric nerve blocks in children. *Br J Anaesth*. 2005;95(2):226–230.
2. Yarwood J, Berrill A. Nerve blocks of the anterior abdominal wall. *Contin Ed Anaesth Crit Care Pain*. 2010;10(6):182–186.
3. Abdellatif AA. Ultrasound-guided ilioinguinal/iliohypogastric nerve blocks versus caudal block for postoperative analgesia in children undergoing unilateral groin surgery. *Saudi J Anaesth*. 2012;6(4):367–372.
4. Dalens B. Lower extremity nerve blocks in pediatric patients. *Tech Reg Anesth Pain Manage*. 2003;7(1):32–47.
5. Van Schoor AN, Boon JM, Bosenberg AT, et al. Anatomical considerations of the pediatric ilioinguinal/iliohypogastric nerve block. *Paediatr Anaesth*. 2005;15(5):371–377.

6. Willschke H, Bösenberg A, Marhofer P, et al. Ultrasonographic-guided ilioinguinal/iliohypogastric nerve block in pediatric anesthesia: what is the optimal volume? *Anesth Analg*. 2006;102(6):1680–1684.
7. Chapman AK, Aucott SW, Gilmore MM, et al. Absorption and tolerability of aqueous chlorhexidine gluconate used for skin antisepsis prior to catheter insertion in preterm neonates. *J Perinatol*. 2013;33(10):768–771.
8. Gofeld M, Christakis M. Sonographically guided ilioinguinal nerve block. *J Ultrasound Med*. 2006;25(12):1571–1575.
9. Neal JM, Mulroy MF, Weinberg GL. American Society of Regional Anesthesia and Pain Medicine checklist for managing local anesthetic systemic toxicity: 2012 version. *Reg Anesth Pain Med*. 2012;37(1):16–18.
10. Abdellatif AA. Ultrasound-guided ilioinguinal/iliohypogastric nerve blocks versus caudal block for postoperative analgesia in children undergoing unilateral groin surgery. *Saudi J Anaesth*. 2012;6(4):367–372.

**8.** Ilioinguinal and Iliohypogastric Nerve Blocks

# Chapter 9

# Transversus Abdominis Plane and Rectus Sheath Blocks

*Natalea Johnson and Jorge A. Pineda*

# Introduction

Truncal peripheral nerve blocks are utilized for supplemental analgesia for abdominal surgeries by providing local anesthesia to the anterior abdominal wall. These blocks are adjuvants because they will not block visceral pain.

For the transversus abdominis plane (TAP) block, an ultrasound probe is traditionally placed in the mid-axillary line between the lower costal margin and the iliac crest, although sometimes this block is performed closer to the surgical site. The three abdominal muscle layers—external oblique, internal oblique, and transversus abdominis—are identified. The needle is inserted under direct ultrasound guidance, and local anesthetic is deposited between the fascial planes of the internal oblique muscle and transversus abdominis muscle.

For a rectus sheath block, the probe is placed slightly lateral to the umbilicus. The aponeurosis of the external oblique muscle, internal oblique muscle, and transversus abdominis muscle converge and are identified as the hyperechoic line at the lateral border of rectus muscle. This aponeurosis encircles the rectus muscle to form an anterior and posterior sheath. The needle is then inserted under direct ultrasound visualization with administration of local anesthetic between the posterior border of the rectus muscle and the posterior fascial plane.

# Clinical Applications

The clinical application for a TAP block is to provide analgesia to the skin, muscles, and parietal peritoneum of the abdominal wall. The TAP block reliably provides analgesia to the lower abdominal wall in the T10–L1 distribution. Rectus sheath blocks anesthetize the terminal branches of the lower thoracic intercostal nerves and provide midline analgesia from the xiphoid process to the umbilicus. Surgical indications for TAP blocks include laparotomies, laparoscopies, inguinal hernia repairs, and appendectomies. Rectus sheath block indications include midline surgeries such as single-port appendectomies and umbilical hernia repairs. A single injection will only provide unilateral analgesia; bilateral blocks are required for bilateral coverage. TAP block analgesia is only consistent below the umbilicus, but coverage up to T7 can be accomplished with subcostal approaches or administration of larger local anesthetic volumes.[1,2]

# Contraindications

Contraindications for the TAP or rectus sheath blocks include patient or parental refusal and skin infection at the needle insertion point. A relative contraindication is coagulopathy.

# Critical Anatomy

Innervation of the anterior abdominal wall arises from the anterior rami of the T7–L1 spinal nerves with terminal branches, including the intercostal, subcostal, iliohypogastric, and ilioinguinal nerves, traveling between the internal oblique muscle and the transversus abdominis muscle.

# Setup

## Equipment

- 22- to 25-gauge echogenic regional block needle
- Ultrasound machine with linear probe array and sterile probe cover or sterile occlusive dressing to cover the probe
- Sterile ultrasound gel
- Sterile gloves
- Sterile preparation solution

- Sterile towels or other sterile drape
- 20% intralipid readily available

> **WARNING!!** Alcohol-based skin preparation solutions are a potential fire hazard in the operating room, especially when electrocautery is utilized for the surgical procedure. When using alcohol-based skin prep, do not allow excess preparation solution to pool around or under the patient. Ensure that the alcohol-based skin preparation solution is completely dry and that any excess is wiped away with towels before preparing the patient for surgery.

!! **Potential Complications:** Rare complications include intravascular injection, parietal or intestinal puncture, hematoma, and infection.[3]

***Pearl:*** The parietal peritoneum and abdominal cavity lie posterior to the transversus abdominis muscle. Peristaltic intestinal movement can often be observed.

### Drugs, Dosages, Administration

This is a field block relying on local anesthetic spread to achieve appropriate nerve blockade. The drug used for these procedures is 0.25 mL/kg of 0.25% bupivacaine or ropivacaine, not to exceed recommended maximum local anesthetic doses.[4]

> **WARNING!!** It is important to calculate the allowable total local anesthetic dose by weight and to stay below this maximum dose in order to decrease the risk for local anesthetic systemic toxicity. This calculation should include all local anesthetics, including that given by the surgeon, intravenous (IV) local anesthetic given by the anesthesiologist, and EMLA or subcutaneous lidocaine given before starting an intravenous line.

Before the start of the case, gather all necessary equipment. Based on the patient's body weight, calculate an appropriate dose of local anesthetic and adjuvant (if desired).

>> **Tip on Technique:** It may be useful to gather all supplies on a mobile flat surface, such as a mayo stand, to utilize for equipment setup during the procedure.

> **Caution!** Double-check your patient's allergies before collection of medications and antiseptic solutions.

## Step-by-Step

1. **Prepare before the procedure.** Place standard American Society of Anesthesiologists monitors on the child and then administer a general anesthetic by intravenous or inhalational techniques. Place the intravenous line, if it is not already in situ, and secure the airway for the surgical procedure. The block itself is performed either before or after the surgical procedure.

*Pearl:* Performing the block before the surgical procedure can assist with surgical analgesia, decreasing the need for opioid dosing during the surgery. Some surgeons, however, have the opinion that the fluid injected near the surgical site interferes with surgical visualization and therefore prefer that the block be performed after the completion of the surgery.

2. **Position the patient and prepare the skin.** The child should remain supine with the abdominal region exposed for either the TAP or the rectus sheath nerve block. Identify the relevant landmarks: the umbilicus and the surgical site. Using sterile gloves, prepare a wide circular area of skin on the side on which you are performing the block. Using a sterile prep solution, and clean the area from the anterior-superior iliac spine to the umbilicus.

> **WARNING!!** Chlorhexidine topical solution is contraindicated for use in premature infants or infants younger than 2 months because of the risks for irritation or chemical burn and potential systemic absorption.

3. **Place the ultrasound probe and identify the three layers of muscle.** For the TAP block, place the ultrasound probe horizontally in the mid-axillary line between the subcostal margin and iliac crest (Figure 9.1). Identify the three muscle layers—the external oblique muscle, internal oblique muscle, and transversus abdominis muscle—by sliding the probe medial to lateral or cephalad to caudad to obtain the clearest facial planes (Figure 9.2). The internal oblique muscle is typically the thickest muscle, and the transversus abdominis muscle is typically the thinnest.

For the rectus sheath block, place the probe horizontally at or just lateral to the umbilicus and identify the linea alba and corresponding rectus muscle. Moving the probe laterally illustrates the thinning of the rectus muscle into the thin facial aponeurosis of the external oblique muscle, internal oblique muscle, and transversus abdominis muscle that then blooms into three distinct muscle bundles posteriorly.

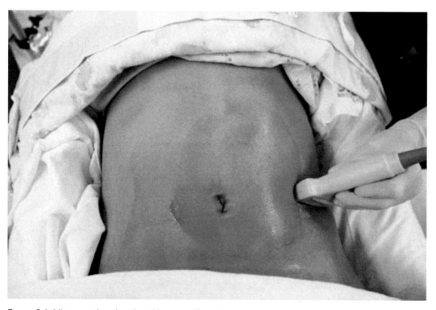

Figure 9.1 Ultrasound probe placed horizontally in the mid-axillary line between the subcostal margin and iliac crest.

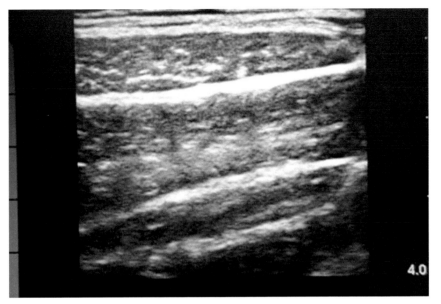

**Figure 9.2** Three muscle layers are identified on ultrasound: external oblique muscle, internal oblique muscle, and transversus abdominis muscle.

If there is difficulty identifying the three layers for a TAP block, scan from midline to lateral until the layers are visualized, as described earlier. Adjustment of the ultrasound depth and gain in order to optimize image quality based on patient's age and habitus may be necessary.

4. **Insert the needle.** For the TAP block, insert the needle under direct ultrasound guidance, with an in-plane approach, to reach the fascial plane separating the internal oblique muscle and the transversus abdominis muscle (Figures 9.3 and 9.4). For the rectus sheath block, insert the needle with an in-plane approach, under direct ultrasound guidance to reach the aponeurosis that is directly superficial to the posterior rectus muscle.

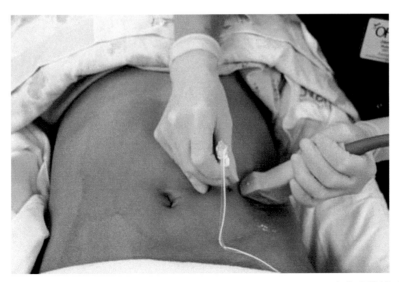

**Figure 9.3** Needle inserted under direct ultrasound guidance, in-plane approach, for TAP block.

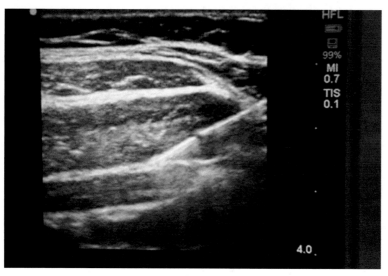

**Figure 9.4** Ultrasound image of needle inserted under direct ultrasound guidance, in-plane approach, for TAP block.

5. **Inject local anesthetic.** Aspirate for blood and, if negative, inject a small amount of local anesthetic to confirm the correct needle position. For the TAP block, visualize hypoechoic local expansion between the internal oblique muscle and transverse abdominis muscle, with the local anesthetic dose pushing the transverse abdominis muscle posteriorly (Figure 9.5).

For the rectus sheath block, the injection of local anesthetic should push the rectus muscle anteriorly, separating it from the posterior fascial layer. Seeing this spread is one sign that the needle tip is not intramuscular. For both blocks, after confirming the correct needle location, inject the local anesthetic dose with intermittent aspiration while under continuous visualization.

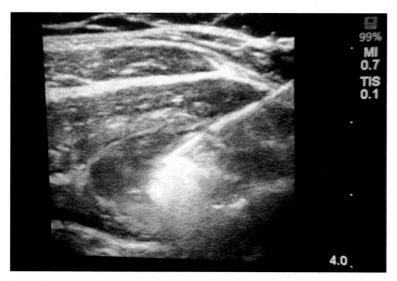

**Figure 9.5** Ultrasound image of hypoechoic local expansion between the internal oblique muscle and transverse abdominis muscle, with the local anesthetic dose pushing the transverse abdominis muscle posteriorly.

## Postoperative Management Considerations

In patients with a functioning nerve block, opioid requirements may be reduced. Caregivers should be warned to expect the need for analgesia to increase as the block slowly "wears off." The sensation over the area blocked will remain decreased for approximately 4 to 6 hours, similar to a caudal block. Caregivers should be told to carefully place their child in a car seat or seat belt so as to avoid injury to the surgical area.

## References

1. Tran TMN, Ivanusic JJ, Hebbard P, Barrington MJ. Determination of spread of injectate after ultrasound-guided transversus abdominis plane block: a cadaveric study. *Br J Anaesth.* 2008;102(1):123–127.
2. Barrington MJ, Ivanusic JJ, Rozen WM, Hebbard P. Spread of injectate after ultrasound-guided subcostal transversus abdominis plane block: a cadaveric study. *Anaesthesia.* 2009;64(7):745–750.
3. Long JB, Birmingham PK, De Oliveira GS Jr, et al. Transversus abdominis plane block in children: a multicenter safety analysis of 1994 cases from the PRAN (Pediatric Regional Anesthesia Network) database. *Anesth Analg.* 2014;119(2):395–399.
4. Santhanam S, Chan VWS. Ultrasound guided transversus abdominis plane block in infants, children and adolescents: a simple procedural guidance for their performance. *Pediatr Anesth.* 2009;19(4):296–299.

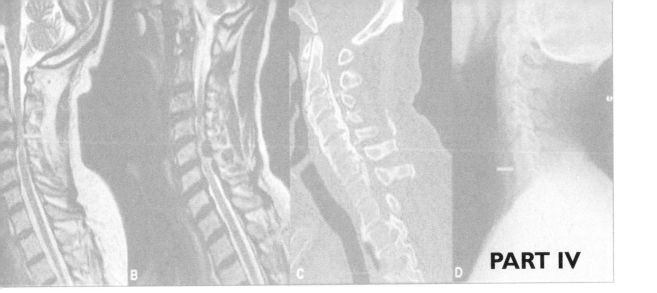

B    C    D

**PART IV**

# RADIOLOGY

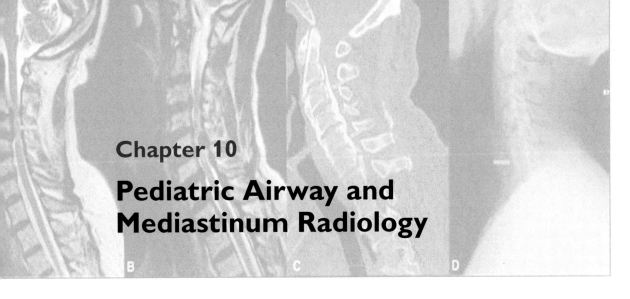

# Chapter 10

# Pediatric Airway and Mediastinum Radiology

*Joshua H. Finkle*

# Airway

## Epiglottitis

Epiglottitis is an acute bacterial infection of the upper airway with prominent edema of the epiglottis and surrounding soft tissues. The infection is classically caused by *Haemophilus influenzae*, a bacterial agent for which there is now routine immunization, leading to a significant decrease in the incidence of epiglottitis in recent decades.[1] Diagnosis is made on lateral radiographs of the neck, which are acquired with a technique to optimize the conspicuity of soft tissue structures. The epiglottis will be enlarged and indistinct, with additional aryepiglottic soft tissue thickening (Figure 10.1).

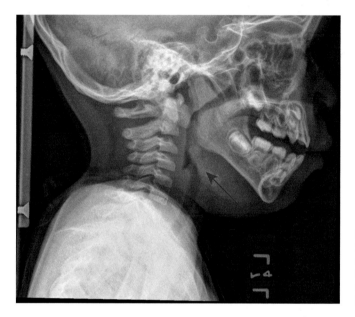

Figure 10.1 Lateral neck radiograph in a child with difficulty breathing shows thickening and indistinctness of the epiglottis (arrow), indicating epiglottitis.

---

**Caution!** The diagnosis is confirmed with direct visualization by laryngoscopy, and urgent intubation may be needed for patients with severe disease.

**Caution!** The radiograph must be obtained in a direct lateral position. If there is rotation, a normal epiglottis may appear abnormally thickened.

---

## Croup

Croup, or viral laryngotracheobronchitis, is a common cause of airway obstruction in children. Croup is most commonly caused by the parainfluenza or influenza virus and, as an upper airway process, leads to the classical clinical symptoms of inspiratory stridor and a characteristic "barking" cough.[2] Croup is a predominantly clinical diagnosis, but a frontal radiograph of the neck may show narrowing and loss of the normal convexity of the subglottic trachea, called the "steeple sign" (Figure 10.2), along with hypopharyngeal distension on the lateral view.

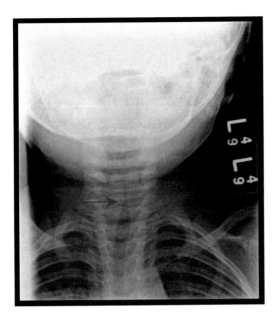

**Figure 10.2** Anterior-posterior soft tissue neck radiograph in a child with stridor shows narrowing and loss of the normal convexity of the subglottic larynx (arrow), called the "steeple sign," suggesting croup.

**Note:** While croup and exudative tracheitis cause bilateral subglottic narrowing, asymmetric or unilateral nodular narrowing may represent a mass lesion such as a subglottic hemangioma. A computed tomography (CT) angiogram can be performed for confirmation if this diagnosis is suspected.

### Exudative Tracheitis
Bacterial tracheitis is another infectious cause of upper airway obstruction in children. Caused by *Staphylococcus, Moraxella, Streptococcus,* or *Haemophilus* species, this infection causes upper airway erosion, mucosal sloughing, and thick mucus production, which can lead to life-threatening airway obstruction.[3] Radiographic findings in exudative tracheitis may overlap with those of croup, with subglottic airway narrowing and possible wall irregularity. Many patients will also show evidence of pneumonia on chest imaging.

### Congenital Tracheomalacia
Tracheomalacia is often due to abnormality of the muscular and cartilaginous supporting tissues of the large airways, which leads to weakness and collapse of the trachea and large bronchi. This presents with variable chronic respiratory symptoms in children with an association with prematurity and other cartilage disorders like relapsing polychondritis. Radiographs and fluoroscopy may show a decrease in tracheal caliber with expiration, although CT is quite sensitive and increasingly used for diagnosis. More than 50% anterior-posterior tracheobronchial collapse on expiration CT images is considered diagnostic (Figure 10.3A and B).[4]

Laryngomalacia represents a similar process in the supraglottic airway and is the most common cause of congenital stridor. Airway fluoroscopy may show collapse of the upper airway during inspiration, although direct laryngoscopy is often the diagnostic procedure of choice.

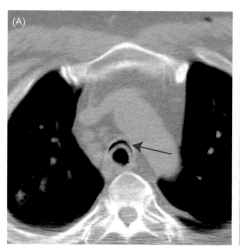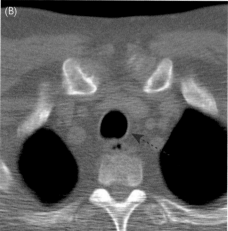

Figure 10.3 Computed tomography image obtained during expiration (**A**) shows marked collapse of the trachea in the anterior-posterior dimension (arrow 1) in a patient with tracheomalacia. On inspiration (**B**), this finding reverses, and the trachea has a normal morphology (arrow 2).

## Obstructive Sleep Apnea

In children, obstructive sleep apnea (OSA) is commonly caused by tonsillar and adenoidal hypertrophy. Other causes include obesity and pharyngeal muscle hypotonia. Cases of moderate or severe tonsillar enlargement can be treated surgically, and imaging is often performed for evaluation. Lateral radiographs of the neck readily demonstrate the size of the adenoids and palatine tonsils (Figure 10.4). Magnetic resonance imaging can also be used for volumetric and dynamic assessment.[5]

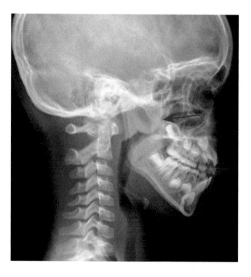

Figure 10.4 Lateral neck radiograph in a child with snoring shows enlarged adenoids (arrow) with resultant narrowing of the nasopharyngeal airway.

## Retropharyngeal Abscess

In the setting of an acute bacterial infection, inflammatory fluid may accumulate in the potential space between the pharynx and vertebral bodies. When a discrete walled-off fluid collection is formed, the process has progressed from retropharyngeal cellulitis to an abscess. Common causative agents are *Streptococcus, Staphylococcus,* and *Haemophilus* species, and most patients are younger than 5 years.[6] A well-positioned lateral radiograph of the neck will demonstrate thickening of the soft tissues between the vertebral bodies and airway (Figure 10.5A and B). In young children, the upper cervical prevertebral soft tissue thickness should be less than half the diameter of the adjacent vertebral body. In suspected cases, contrast-enhanced CT is often performed to confirm and characterize the abscess.

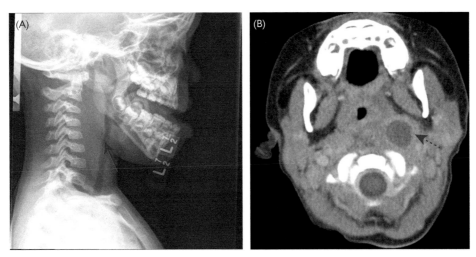

**Figure 10.5** Lateral neck radiograph (**A**) in a child with fever and difficulty swallowing shows enlargement of the prevertebral soft tissues (arrow 1). Computed tomography (**B**) shows a peripherally enhancing collection in the left retropharyngeal space (arrow 2) compatible with an abscess.

## Esophageal Atresia and Tracheoesophageal Fistula

A heterogeneous group of anomalies, esophageal atresia and tracheoesophageal fistula (TEF), may be present in any of several configurations. The most common configuration is esophageal atresia with a fistula between the trachea and the distal esophageal pouch. TEF is highly associated with other congenital anomalies and is part of the VACTERL syndrome (vertebral abnormalities, anal atresia, cardiac abnormalities, tracheoesophageal fistula and/or esophageal atresia, renal agenesis and dysplasia, and limb defects).[7]

| **WARNING!!** | In patients with a tracheoesophageal fistula, positive pressure ventilation, especially at high pressures, can lead to inflation of the stomach and severe, life-threatening impairment of ventilation that, in some cases, can only be resolved by needle decompression of the stomach. |
|---|---|

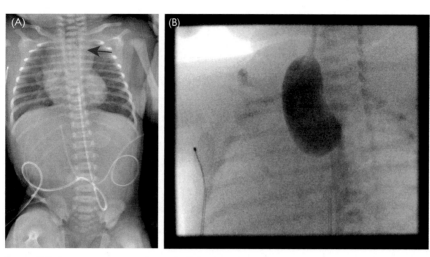

Figure 10.6 Anterior-posterior radiograph of the chest and abdomen (**A**) in a newborn shows a feeding tube with its tip unable to pass much beyond the cervicothoracic junction (arrow), indicating esophageal atresia. Absence of bowel gas in this case rules out a fistula between the trachea and distal esophageal pouch. Fluoroscopic image from an esophagram (**B**) shows contrast pooling within the proximal esophageal pouch.

The radiographic appearance will differ depending on the type of anomaly. In any newborn with esophageal atresia, a feeding tube will be unable to advance beyond the atretic upper portion of the esophagus (Figure 10.6A and B). If there is no distal TEF, there will be an absence of bowel gas because swallowed gas is unable to pass beyond the upper esophagus. If there is a distal TEF, bowel gas may be normal or even increased in the setting of positive pressure ventilation.

## Vascular Impressions on the Trachea and Esophagus

### Double Aortic Arch

Typically, the embryologic right fourth aortic arch regresses, with the left fourth arch remaining as the aortic arch. With a double aortic arch, both fourth arches persist, each usually with its own common carotid and subclavian artery branches. A double aortic arch is a true vascular ring, with the two arch branches completely encasing the trachea and esophagus. A double aortic arch is usually not associated with other congenital anomalies.[8]

Radiographs may show narrowing of the trachea at the level of the aortic arch, with bilateral mediastinal soft tissue suggesting the diagnosis (Figure 10.7A–D). Lateral fluoroscopic evaluation will show a posterior impression on the esophagus and an anterior impression on the trachea. CT angiography can be performed for confirmation and surgical planning.

### Aberrant Right Subclavian Artery

An aberrant right subclavian artery is the most common aortic arch branch variant. The aberrant artery arises as the distalmost branch of the aortic arch and courses to the right posterior to the esophagus. An aberrant right subclavian artery is not a true vascular ring and is usually asymptomatic. However, patients may have associated dysphagia, termed *dysphagia lusoria*.[9] Fluoroscopy will show a posterior impression on the esophagus (Figure 10.8A–D). CT angiography can confirm the diagnosis.

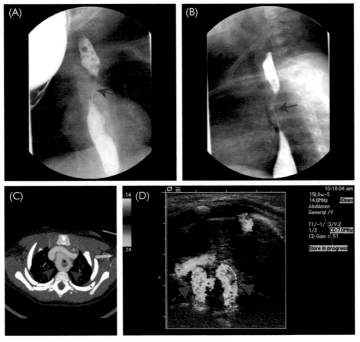

Figure 10.7 Anterior-posterior and lateral fluoroscopic images from an esophagram (**A** and **B**) show esophageal narrowing at the level of the aortic arch (solid arrows). Computed tomography angiogram (**C**) shows the left and right aortic arches (dashed arrows) creating a vascular ring around the esophagus and narrowed trachea. Color Doppler ultrasound (**D**) shows flow within both aortic arches (arrows 3).

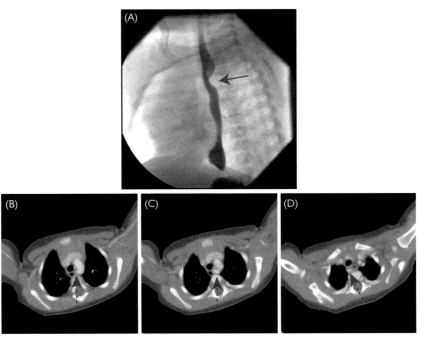

Figure 10.8 Oblique lateral fluoroscopic image from an esophagram (**A**) shows focal extrinsic compression on the posterior esophagus (solid arrow). Axial computed tomography images (**B–D**) show the aberrant right subclavian artery (dashed arrows) coursing posterior to the esophagus.

## Right Aortic Arch with Aberrant Left Subclavian Artery

The two most common configurations with a right aortic arch are mirror-image branching and aberrant left subclavian artery. Right aortic arch with mirror-image branching is the direct mirror image of the typical anatomy and therefore does not create a vascular ring. A right aortic arch with mirror-image branching is strongly associated with other congenital anomalies, including tetralogy of Fallot and truncus arteriosus.

A right-sided aortic arch with an aberrant left subclavian artery is the direct mirror image of a left-sided arch with aberrant right subclavian artery. This anomaly, however, represents a true vascular ring, with the ligamentum arteriosum completing the left side of the ring at the level of the aortic arch. Like a double aortic arch, fluoroscopy will show a posterior impression on the esophagus and an anterior impression on the trachea. CT angiography can be performed for confirmation.

## Pulmonary Sling

The normal pulmonary artery anatomy has the right and left main pulmonary arteries arising directly from the pulmonary trunk and both coursing anterior to the airway and esophagus. In pulmonary sling, the left pulmonary artery arises as a branch of the right and courses leftward between the trachea and esophagus. Although this is not a true ring, local tracheal compression can lead to airway obstructive symptoms.[10] Lateral view fluoroscopy will show an impression anterior to the esophagus and posterior to the trachea (Figure 10.9A–D). A CT can confirm the diagnosis.

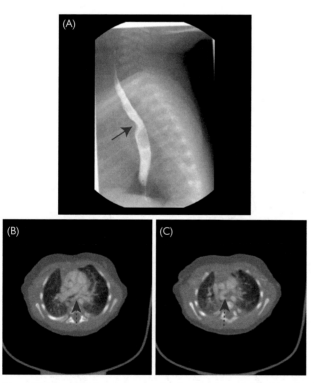

Figure 10.9 Lateral fluoroscopic image from an esophagram (**A**) shows focal extrinsic compression on the anterior esophagus (arrow 1). Computed tomography scans (**B–D**) show the left pulmonary artery arising from the right and coursing leftward between the trachea and esophagus (arrow 2). This is a pulmonary sling.

## Esophageal and Tracheal Foreign Bodies

Foreign bodies, if they are composed of a dense enough material, can only be directly visualized on radiographs. Ingested foreign bodies in the chest may be within the esophagus or trachea (Figure 10.10). Coins are the most commonly seen ingested radiopaque foreign body in children (Figure 10.11A and B).[11]

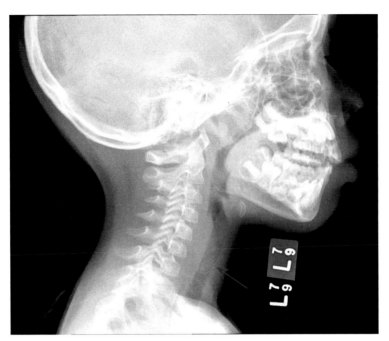

Figure 10.10  Lateral neck radiograph shows a sunflower seed (arrow) within the trachea of a child.

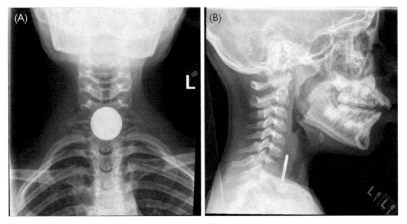

Figure 10.11  Anterior-posterior (**A**) and lateral (**B**) views of the neck show a metallic disc (a coin) at the level of the thoracic inlet. The lateral view clearly shows that the coin is located in the esophagus and not the trachea (lucent area anterior to the coin).

Ingested button batteries may lead to tissue damage due to a combination of electrical discharge, leakage of corrosives, and direct pressure. These foreign bodies are therefore considered for emergent endoscopic retrieval, particularly if still in the esophagus at the time of imaging. Button batteries can be distinguished from coins on radiographs by a faint lucent rim near the edge of the battery (Figure 10.12).

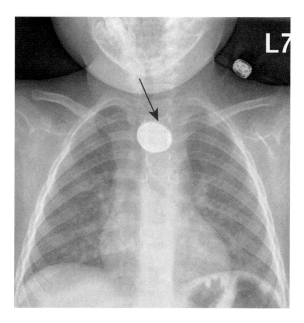

Figure 10.12 Anterior-posterior radiograph of the chest shows a metallic disc near the thoracic inlet. In this case, a lucent rim (arrow) indicates that this is a button battery and not a coin.

### Bronchial Foreign Body

Small pieces of food are common bronchial foreign bodies and are usually radiolucent and therefore not directly visualized on radiographs. Potentially severe airway obstruction necessitates prompt diagnosis. A standard frontal chest radiograph may show hyperinflation of the affected lung because the foreign body can lead to partial airway obstruction and air trapping. However, a chest radiograph may be completely normal. In this case, left and right decubitus views of the

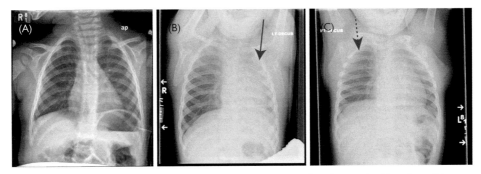

Figure 10.13 Anterior-posterior radiograph of the chest (**A**) appears relatively normal, with perhaps slight hyperexpansion of the right lung. A left lateral decubitus view (**B**) shows normal partial atelectasis of the depended left lung (arrow 1) while the right lung remains aerated. On right lateral decubitus view (**C**), the dependent right lung remains expanded (arrow 2), indicating (abnormal) air trapping. This patient had a peanut lodged in the right mainstem bronchus.

chest can be obtained. In a normal patient, the dependent lung will show partial atelectasis. In a patient with a bronchial foreign body, however, the affected lung will remain inflated in both dependent and nondependent positions (Figure 10.13A–C).[13]

## Mediastinum

### Normal Thymus

The thymus resides in the anterior mediastinum, has a highly variable appearance in young children (a normal thymus may be quite large in children), and should not be mistaken for a mass or other abnormality. On radiographs, the thymus may present as a "sail sign," a triangular soft tissue density indicating thymic tissue sitting on the minor fissure (Figure 10.14A and B). On ultrasound, the thymus has a starry-sky appearance similar to liver parenchyma.[14]

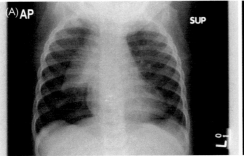
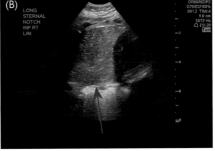

Figure 10.14 Anterior-posterior radiograph of the chest (**A**) shows a triangular soft tissue density along the right mediastinal border. This is a "sail sign" appearance of a normal thymus. On ultrasound (**B**), the thymus (arrow) shows a speckled "starry-sky" appearance.

**Caution!** In children under positive pressure ventilation, the thymus may be seen "lifted" off the underlying mediastinum with gas directly beneath the thymus. This is termed the "spinnaker sail sign" and is NOT a normal appearance of the thymus but rather an indication of pneumomediastinum (Figure 10.15).[15]

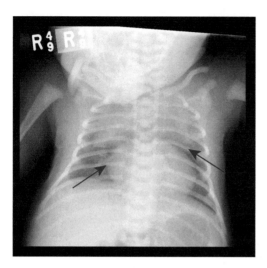

**Figure 10.15** Anterior-posterior radiograph of the chest shows elevation of the thymus, with lucency between thymic tissue and the upper borders of the heart bilaterally (arrows). This is the "spinnaker sail sign," indicating pneumomediastinum.

**Pearl:** In cancer patients following completion of chemotherapy, the thymus may significantly increase in volume. This physiologic process is called thymic rebound (Figure 10.16A and B) and should not be confused with mediastinal pathology.

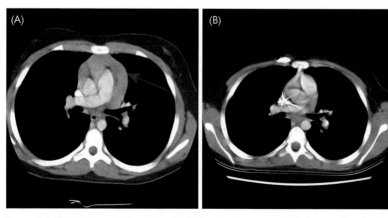

**Figure 10.16** Chest computed tomography (CT) scan of a teenager (**A**) shows soft tissue in the anterior mediastinum (arrow) compatible with an enlarged thymus. This patient had recently finished chemotherapy for leukemia, and CT performed 2 months earlier (**B**) (while still undergoing chemotherapy) showed essentially no thymic tissue. This represents the normal physiologic process of thymic rebound.

## Mediastinal Masses

Mediastinal masses can arise from any of the various tissue types residing in the mediastinum. These masses are categorized by location as arising from the anterior, middle, or posterior mediastinum. Localization helps with narrowing the differential diagnosis and guiding treatment options.[16]

> **Caution!** A mediastinal mass can cause complete obstruction of the trachea or bronchi and the inability to ventilate when general anesthesia is administered, especially when a muscle relaxant is given.

### Anterior Mediastinal Masses

Lymphoma is the most common cause of mediastinal mass in children and often presents as a large anterior mass. The primary differential for an anterior mediastinal mass includes germ cell tumors and thymic tumors.[17] Radiographs can help localize a mass to the anterior mediastinum. On frontal radiographs, there may be loss of the normal anterior structure borders, including the cardiophrenic angles and ascending aorta (Figure 10.17A–C). Because hilar markings (central airways and pulmonary vessels—middle mediastinal structures) are intact, they may be visualized through the mass. The lateral view may show abnormal soft tissue within the normal retrosternal clear space. CT is often performed for confirmation and further characterization of the mass.

### Middle Mediastinal Masses

Most middle mediastinal masses are developmental cystic abnormalities of the embryologic foregut. Lymphadenopathy, pericardial cysts, and lipomas make up most of the remaining middle mediastinal masses.[18] Radiographs may show distortion of the normal middle mediastinal structures, including the paratracheal stripes, anterior-posterior window, and hila

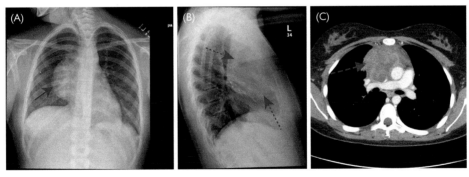

Figure 10.17  Posterior-anterior (**A**) and lateral (**B**) radiographs show a mass within the right aspect of the mediastinum (arrow 1). There is loss of the normal right heart border, and the lateral view shows loss of the normal retrosternal clear space (arrows 2), indicating anterior location of the mass. Additionally, the right hilar vasculature (a middle mediastinal structure) is clearly visualized through the mass, indicating that the middle mediastinum is not involved. Chest computed tomography (**C**) shows the anterior mediastinal mass (arrow 3), which was lymphoma.

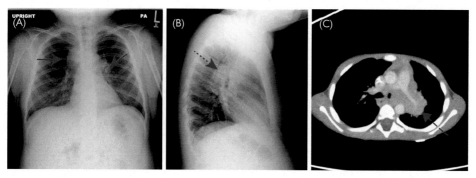

**Figure 10.18** Posterior-anterior chest radiograph (**A**) shows abnormal mediastinal soft tissue bilaterally (arrows 1). On the lateral view (**B**), the soft tissue is seen surrounding the mainstem bronchi, the "doughnut sign." (arrow 2) Chest computed tomography (**C**) shows soft tissue encasing the central pulmonary arteries (arrow 3). This patient had lymphoma with significant hilar lymphadenopathy.

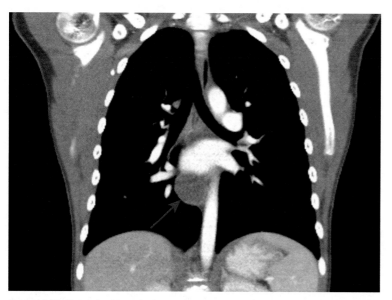

**Figure 10.19** Coronal computed tomography scan of the chest, abdomen, and pelvis shows a fluid-density mass (arrow) within the middle mediastinum compatible with a duplication cyst.

(Figures 10.18A–C and 10.19). The lateral view may show a "doughnut sign," with soft tissue surrounding the hilar bronchovascular structures. CT is frequently performed for further characterization.

**Note:** A vascular lesion such as one of the arch anomalies described in the previous section can mimic a middle mediastinal mass.

## Posterior Mediastinal Masses

Many tissues are present in the posterior mediastinum, including nerves, lymph nodes, vessels, and bones. The most common group of posterior mediastinal masses are neurogenic in origin

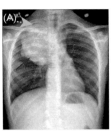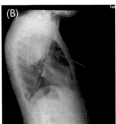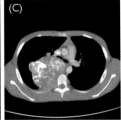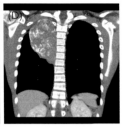

**Figure 10.20** Posterior-anterior (**A**) and lateral (**B**) chest radiographs show a large mass along the right medi-astinum (solid red arrows). The posterior-anterior view (**A**) shows the soft tissue of the mass extending above the level of the clavicle, the "cervicothoracic sign," (dashed green arrow) indicating a posterior mediastinal or-igin of this mass. Computed tomography (**C** and **D**) shows that this large posterior mediastinal mass contains calcifications, strongly suggestive of neuroblastoma, the diagnosis in this case.

and include neuroblastoma, neurofibroma, neurenteric cyst, and schwannoma. Chest wall prim-itive neuroectodermal tumors, Ewing sarcoma, and extramedullary hematopoiesis may also present as one or multiple posterior mediastinal masses.[19] On radiographs, loss of the distinct paravertebral stripe indicates posterior location. Additionally, any mediastinal mass extending above the clavicle is most likely in the posterior mediastinum (Figure 10.20A–D).

# References

1. Shah RK, Roberson DW, Jones DT. Epiglottitis in the *Hemophilus influenzae* type B vaccine era: changing trends. *Laryngoscope.* 2004;114(3):557–560.
2. Leung AK, Kellner JD, Johnson DW. Viral croup: a current perspective. *J Pediatr Health Care.* 2004;18(6):297–301.
3. Lee JK, Yoon TM, Oh SE, Lim SC. Treatment of exudative tracheitis with acute airway ob-struction under jet ventilation. *Otolaryngol Head Neck Surg.* 2008;139(4):606–607.
4. Lee EY, Tracy DA, Bastos M, et al. Expiratory volumetric MDCT evaluation of air trapping in pediatric patients with and without tracheomalacia. *AJR Am J Roentgenol.* 2010;194(5):1210–1215.
5. Donnelly LF, Casper KA, Chen B. Correlation on cine MR imaging of size of adenoid and palatine tonsils with degree of upper airway motion in asymptomatic sedated children. *AJR Am J Roentgenol.* 2002;179(2):503–508.
6. Craig FW, Schunk JE. Retropharyngeal abscess in children: clinical presentation, utility of imaging, and current management. *Pediatrics.* 2003;111(6 Pt 1):1394–1398.
7. Stoll C, Alembik Y, Dott B, Roth MP. Associated malformations in patients with esophageal atresia. *Eur J Med Genet.* 2009;52(5):287–290.
8. Bonnard A, Auber F, Fourcade L, et al. Vascular ring abnormalities: a retrospective study of 62 cases. *J Pediatr Surg.* 2003;38(4):539–543.
9. Woods RK, Sharp RJ, Holcomb GW 3rd, et al. Vascular anomalies and tracheoesophageal compression: a single institution's 25-year experience. *Ann Thorac Surg.* 2001;72(2):434–438; discussion 438–439.
10. Newman B, Cho Y. Left pulmonary artery sling: anatomy and imaging. *Semin Ultrasound CT MR.* 2010;31(2):158–170.
11. Silva AB, Muntz HR, Clary R. Utility of conventional radiography in the diagnosis and management of pediatric airway foreign bodies. *Ann Otol Rhinol Laryngol.* 1998;107(10 Pt 1):834–838.

12. Schlesinger AE, Crowe JE. Sagittal orientation of ingested coins in the esophagus in children. *AJR Am J Roentgenol.* 2011;196(3):670–672.
13. Svedstrom E, Puhakka H, Kero P. How accurate is chest radiography in the diagnosis of tracheobronchial foreign bodies in children? *Pediatr Radiol.* 1989;19(8):520–522.
14. Nasseri F, Eftekhari F. Clinical and radiologic review of the normal and abnormal thymus: pearls and pitfalls. *Radiographics.* 2010;30(2):413–428.
15. Bullaro FM, Bartoletti SC. Spontaneous pneumomediastinum in children: a literature review. *Pediatr Emerg Care.* 2007;23(1):28–30.
16. Lee EY. Evaluation of non-vascular mediastinal masses in infants and children: an evidence-based practical approach. *Pediatr Radiol.* 2009;39(Suppl 2):S184–S190.
17. Tomiyama N, Honda O, Tsubamoto M, et al. Anterior mediastinal tumors: diagnostic accuracy of CT and MRI. *Eur J Radiol.* 2009;69(2):280–288.
18. Coley BD, Caffey J. *Caffey's pediatric diagnostic imaging.* 12th ed. Philadelphia,: Saunders; 2013.
19. Kawashima A, Fishman EK, Kuhlman JE. CT and MR evaluation of posterior mediastinal masses. *Crit Rev Diagn Imaging.* 1992;33(4):311–367.

**10.** Pediatric Airway and Mediastinum Radiology

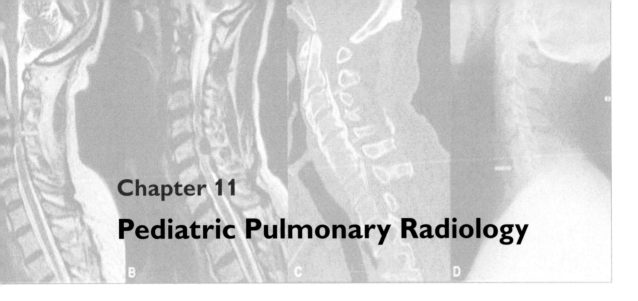

# Chapter 11

# Pediatric Pulmonary Radiology

*Joshua H. Finkle*

# Neonatal Chest

## Meconium Aspiration

When meconium is passed in utero, the fetus may inhale meconium-stained amniotic fluid. This causes a chemical pneumonitis that can lead to respiratory failure. Post-term birth and prolonged labor are risk factors.[1] Radiographs will show patchy and "rope-like" opacities throughout the lungs (Figure 11.1). There also may be pleural effusions.

**Note:** This is an obstructive process of small airways, and lung volumes are often increased. Pneumothorax is a possible complication.

## Transient Tachypnea of the Newborn

Also called "wet lung disease," transient tachypnea of the newborn (TTN) results from retained fetal fluid within the lungs. This process may lead to respiratory distress, which typically resolves within hours to days of birth.[2] Radiographs will show an interstitial edema pattern of lung opacities with small pleural effusions, classically seen as a small amount of fluid in the minor fissure (Figure 11.2). These imaging findings should resolve within 48 hours.

**Note:** Fetal lung fluid is cleared in the perinatal period in response to the physical stresses related to birth. Babies born by cesarean delivery do not undergo these normal stresses and are therefore at higher risk for TTN.

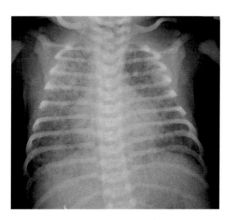

Figure 11.1 Anterior-posterior radiograph of the chest in a term neonate born with meconium-stained amniotic fluid shows coarse patchy opacities throughout both lungs indicating meconium aspiration.

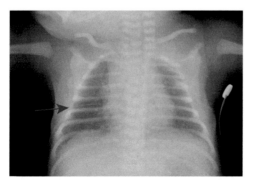

Figure 11.2 Anterior-posterior radiograph of the chest in a neonate with respiratory distress shows mild perihilar and basilar opacities with a small amount of fluid seen within the minor fissure (arrow). Symptoms and radiographic findings resolved within 24 hours, indicating transient tachypnea of the newborn as the diagnosis.

## Respiratory Distress Syndrome

Respiratory distress syndrome (RDS), also called hyaline membrane disease, results from a deficiency of lung surfactant at birth, which leads to diffuse alveolar collapse and respiratory failure. Although some surfactant is expressed as early as 20 weeks, mature surfactant does not usually form until about 34 to 35 weeks of gestation, so babies born earlier than 35 weeks are at much higher risk for developing RDS.[3] Radiographs will show diffuse hazy and granular lung opacities (Figure 11.3). Lung volumes will be decreased, reflecting the underlying pathology of diffuse atelectasis, although intubated patients may have normal or even increased lung volumes.

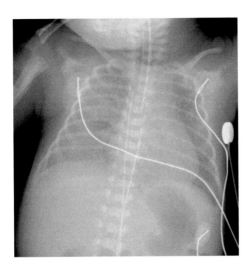

Figure 11.3 Anterior-posterior radiograph of the chest and abdomen in a premature neonate with respiratory distress shows diffuse hazy and granular lung opacities of respiratory distress syndrome.

## Pulmonary Interstitial Emphysema

Pulmonary interstitial emphysema (PIE) is a complication of respiratory distress syndrome and positive pressure ventilation. In the setting of poor lung compliance, high pressure air will rupture small airways and dissect through interstitial tissue and lymphatics. When this occurs, it usually happens within the first week of life.[4] Radiographs will show linear or cystic lucencies extending from the hila (Figure 11.4). Findings may be unilateral or bilateral. Lung volumes may be increased.

**Note:** Gas may escape into adjacent spaces, leading to pneumothorax, pneumomediastinum, or pneumopericardium.

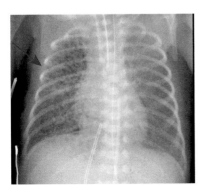

Figure 11.4 Anterior-posterior radiograph of the chest and abdomen in an intubated premature neonate shows small cystic and linear lucencies throughout the right lung (arrow), which appear to radiate from the hilum, compatible with pulmonary interstitial emphysema. The left lung shows the underlying findings of respiratory distress syndrome.

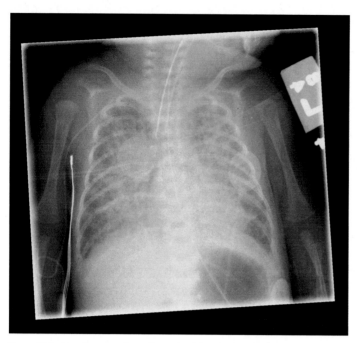

**Figure 11.5** Anterior-posterior radiograph of the chest in a premature neonate who has been undergoing positive pressure ventilation for more than 2 months shows coarse perihilar opacities and scattered areas of scarring, compatible with chronic lung disease of prematurity.

## Bronchopulmonary Dysplasia

Bronchopulmonary dysplasia (BPD), also called chronic lung disease (CLD) of prematurity, is a complication related to chronic positive pressure ventilation of immature lungs during the neonatal period. The pathologic process is complex but involves chronic vascular and small airway damage, resulting in fibroproliferative changes.[5] Radiographic features are highly variable and include scattered coarse peribronchial opacities with areas of scarring or atelectasis as well as hyperinflated, cystic-appearing regions (Figure 11.5).

## Persistent Pulmonary Hypertension

Persistent pulmonary hypertension (PPH) results from a delay in the complex transition from fetal to newborn pulmonary circulation; pulmonary vascular resistance remains high, and blood is shunted through patent physiologic shunts, including the foramen ovale and ductus arteriosus.[6] Imaging features are non-specific, but right-sided cardiac enlargement may be seen on radiography.

## Neonatal Pneumonia

Exposure to bacterial pathogens in utero or during delivery can result in pneumonia. The most common organisms include *Escherichia coli* and *Streptococcus* species. Viruses may also cause neonatal pneumonia, including direct exposure to herpes simplex virus (HSV) during birth and congenital infection with cytomegalovirus (CMV).[7]

Imaging findings are quite variable and may mimic those of transient tachypnea of the newborn or respiratory distress syndrome. In particular, infection with group B *Streptococcus* species, which is screened for during prenatal care, gives a diffuse granular appearance similar to respiratory distress syndrome.

> **Caution!** If a term infant has persistent imaging findings typical of RDS, pneumonia must be considered in the differential diagnosis.

### Congenital Diaphragmatic Hernia

Congenital diaphragmatic hernia (CDH) is a result of the failure of normal fusion of the pleuroperitoneal canals during diaphragm development, which occurs around week 8 of gestation. Imaging findings and management of CDH are discussed in detail in Chapter 19 "Anesthesia for Congenital Diaphragmatic Hernia Repair in Infants" in the companion book to this volume, titled "Pediatric Anesthesia Procedures" published by Oxford University Press.

## Congenital Lung Anomalies

Numerous entities comprise the spectrum of congenital lung anomalies. Each entity is defined by its predominant abnormal tissue type. For example, arteriovenous malformations (AVMs) are predominantly vascular abnormalities, and congenital pulmonary airway malformations (CPAMs) are considered parenchymal abnormalities. In this section, congenital lobar overinflation, bronchopulmonary sequestration, and CPAM are reviewed; however, scimitar syndrome, foregut duplication cyst, pulmonary hypoplasia, and bronchial atresia are other entities that may fall within this spectrum. Hybrid lesions, which show features of multiple malformations,[8] are also very common.

### Congenital Lobar Overinflation

Congenital lobar overinflation (CLO), also called congenital lobar emphysema, is predominantly an airway component abnormality. This is frequently caused by a narrowed or absent lobar bronchus, which leads to air trapping. Extrinsic narrowing by a mediastinal mass or large vessel is common, and there is an association with local bronchial atresia.[9] Radiographs and computed tomography (CT) scans will show an area of hyperlucent lung with a lobar or segmental distribution. The affected lung will have relatively decreased vascularity, and the underlying abnormal bronchus may be directly visualized (Figure 11.6A and B).

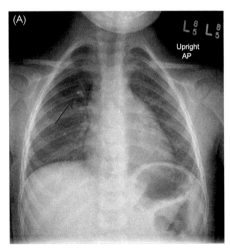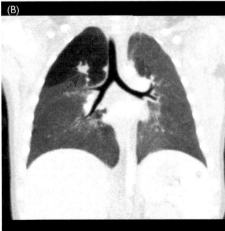

**Figure 11.6** Anterior-posterior radiograph of the chest (**A**) shows relative lucency of the right upper lobe with a small dense focus in the right upper perihilar region (solid arrow). Coronal chest computed tomography (**B**) shows the abnormal hyperinflated right upper lobe as well as the adjacent abnormal bronchus (dashed arrow). This is congenital lobar hyperinflation.

## Bronchopulmonary Sequestration

A bronchopulmonary sequestration is an area of abnormal lung tissue that does not connect with the tracheobronchial tree. Accordingly, these lesions are usually not aerated. Sequestrations are defined by prominent feeding blood flow from the systemic arterial circulation.

**Note:** Sequestrations are categorized as either intralobar or extralobar based on the pleural covering: Intralobar sequestrations do not have their own pleura, whereas extralobar sequestrations are covered by a separate pleural layer and may even be located below the diaphragm.[10]

Contrast-enhanced CT will show a soft tissue mass corresponding to the sequestration with a prominent feeding systemic artery, often a direct branch off the aorta (Figure 11.7).

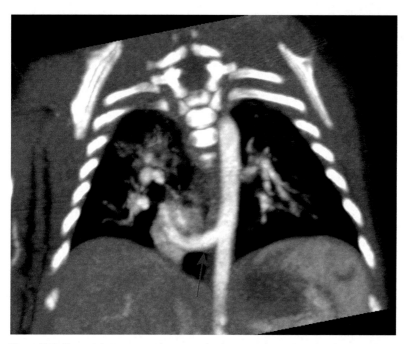

**Figure 11.7** Coronal chest computed tomography shows a soft tissue mass within the right lower lobe. A large feeding artery arising directly from the aorta (arrow) indicates that this mass is a bronchopulmonary sequestration.

## Congenital Pulmonary Airway Malformation

Previously called congenital cystic adenomatoid malformation (CCAM), CPAM is characterized by a localized area of multiple cysts and/or noncystic masses that communicate with an abnormal airway and lack normal cartilaginous support. In contrast to sequestration, CPAMs classically retain feeding vasculature through pulmonary arteries and drain through the pulmonary venous circulation. CPAMs are categorized by the number and size of cysts in the lesion.[11]

Radiographic appearance is highly variable, but a localized region of lung parenchyma containing multiple air-filled cysts is highly suggestive (Figure 11.8). There may also be fluid-filled cysts, particularly if the CPAM is superinfected or solid parenchyma is associated with the lesion.

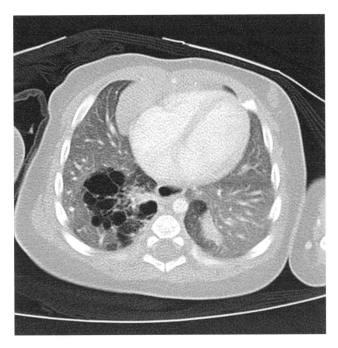

Figure 11.8 Multiple air-filled cysts of varying sizes localized to an area of the right lower lobe are diagnostic of a congenital pulmonary airway malformation.

# Lung Tumors

### Pleuropulmonary Blastoma

Pleuropulmonary blastoma (PPB) is a potentially malignant embryonal tumor originating from the lung. This rare tumor contains primitive mesenchyma as well as fibrous, muscular, and cartilaginous tissue. These tumors may arise within cystic pulmonary lesions, and there is thought to be some overlap between subtypes of pleuropulmonary blastoma and congenital pulmonary airway malformation.[12] Imaging shows a solid or cystic mass within the lung parenchyma with variable enhancement of the solid components (Figure 11.9A–C). In many cases, imaging may be indistinguishable from a congenital pulmonary airway malformation. Other malignant primary lung tumors, including bronchogenic carcinoma and carcinoid tumor, are very rare in children.

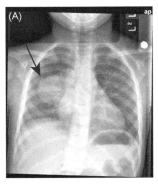
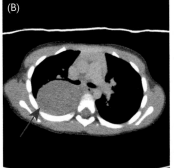
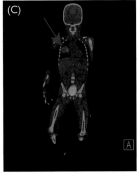

Figure 11.9 Anterior-posterior chest radiograph (**A**), chest computed tomography (**B**), and coronal whole-body positron emission tomography–computed tomography (**C**) show a large hypermetabolic right chest mass arising from the posterior pleura or posterior aspect of the lung (arrows). This is a rare case of pleuropulmonary blastoma.

# Infections

## Pneumonia

Pulmonary bacterial infections are relatively common. The most common agents vary by age group, with *Streptococcus*, *Mycoplasma*, and *Chlamydia* species being common causes of community-acquired pneumonia among multiple age groups. Radiographs will show alveolar consolidation in a lobar or segmental distribution (Figure 11.10A and B). There may be a pleural effusion.

> **WARNING!!** In children younger than 8 years, pneumonia may present as a round mass-like area of consolidation (Figure 11.11A and B). It is important not to mistake round pneumonia for a pulmonary or mediastinal mass!

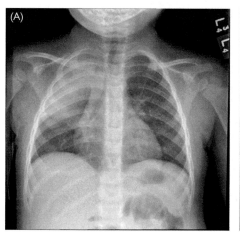 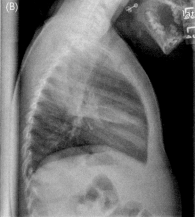

**Figure 11.10** Anterior-posterior (**A**) and lateral (**B**) radiographs of the chest in a child with fever and cough show alveolar air space consolidation in the right upper lobe, compatible with bacterial pneumonia.

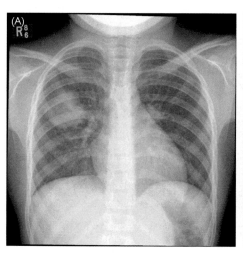 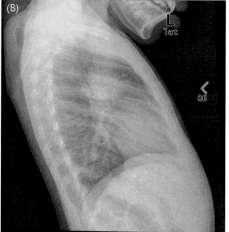

**Figure 11.11** Anterior-posterior (**A**) and lateral (**B**) radiographs of the chest show a round mass-like area of consolidation in the right upper lobe. This was round pneumonia and resolved after antibiotic therapy.

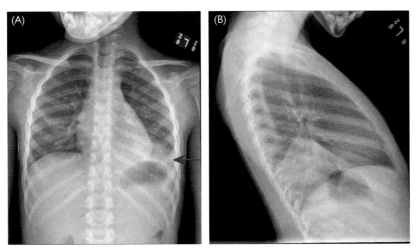

Figure 11.12 The left lower lobe air space consolidation in this patient with pneumonia is difficult to directly visualize on the Anterior-posterior radiograph of the chest (**A**), but complete loss of the normal left diaphragm silhouette (arrow) is the classic imaging feature. The lateral view (**B**) clearly delineates the consolidated left lower lobe.

> **Caution!** Retrocardiac (left lower lobe) consolidation may be difficult to visualize directly on a frontal radiograph (Figure 11.12A and B). Loss of the normal diaphragmatic silhouette is a useful clue, and remember to always look at the lateral view if available.

### Viral Bronchiolitis

Infections by viruses are very common and are typically transmitted by air droplet inhalation. In young children, viral infections cause airway swelling and secretions, leading to an obstructive-type bronchiolitis.[13] Radiographs classically show increased lung volumes, peribronchial soft tissue thickening, and scattered areas of atelectasis (Figure 11.13A and B).

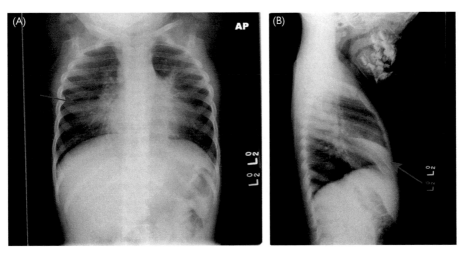

Figure 11.13 Anterior-posterior (**A**) and lateral (**B**) radiographs of the chest in a child with cough and wheezing show perihilar and peribronchial soft tissue prominence as well as scattered areas of atelectasis (arrows), compatible with viral bronchiolitis.

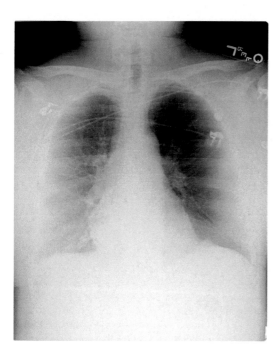

Figure 11.14 Anterior-posterior radiograph of the chest in a young adult shows relative lucency and mild vascular paucity of the left lung compared with the right. This patient had bronchiolitis obliterans involving the left lung during childhood. The resultant chronic findings are called Swyer-James syndrome.

**Pearl:** This pattern of findings is similar to that of airway hyperreactivity typically seen in older children with asthma.

**Note:** In rare cases following bronchiolitis obliterans, a patient may develop chronic imaging findings of unilateral small lung volumes and hyperlucency involving the affected lung (Figure 11.14) which can be seen into adulthood. This sequela is termed Swyer-James-MacLeod syndrome.[14]

## Genetic Disorders

### Sickle Cell Acute Chest Syndrome

Nearly half of all patients with sickle cell disease will at some point develop an illness characterized by fevers, chest pain, and pulmonary opacities on imaging. This is termed acute chest syndrome (ACS). The underlying cause is largely unknown and is thought to be related in part to small vessel infarcts or infection, particularly with viral agents.[15] ACS is characterized by a new alveolar opacity, which may be unilateral or bilateral and is usually in the lower lobes (Figure 11.15). Atelectasis and pleural effusions can also be seen, and scarring may persist after resolution, particularly in patients with repeated episodes of ACS.

**Note:** If not provided in the history, other imaging findings of sickle cell disease, including cardiomegaly and diffuse osseous changes, are useful in making this diagnosis.

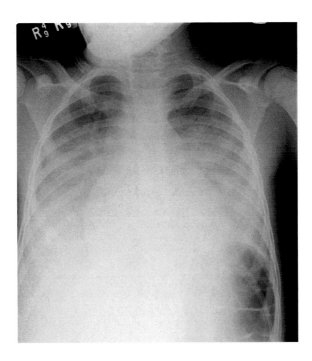

**Figure 11.15** Anterior-posterior radiograph of the chest in a patient with sickle cell disease and acute chest pain shows extensive air space opacities involving both lower lobes, compatible with acute chest syndrome. As is common for this syndrome, the radiographic findings appeared and resolved rapidly. Cardiomegaly is a radiographic clue to the patient's underlying sickle cell disease.

## Cystic Fibrosis

> **WARNING!!** Hemoptysis is a common complication of CF, and massive hemoptysis may lead to asphyxiation. This is an emergency that can be treated with imaging-guided bronchial artery embolization.

Cystic fibrosis (CF) is the most common lethal genetic disease in the United States. Inherited in an autosomal recessive pattern, the disease most commonly involves a mutation of the cystic fibrosis transmembrane conductance regulator *(CFTR)* gene and leads to abnormal production of fluids throughout the body, including airway mucus and digestive fluids. Impaired clearance of abnormally thick airway mucus leads to recurrent bacterial infections and progressive bronchiectasis and mucus plugging.[16] Radiologic gastrointestinal findings of cystic fibrosis are discussed in Chapter 12.

Classic imaging findings in cystic fibrosis include perihilar and apical predominant tubular bronchiectasis with mucus plugging and bronchial wall thickening. Bronchiectasis can be quite severe as the disease progresses (Figure 11.16A–C). Frequently, there is also evidence of acute bronchiolitis, including tree-in-bud and nodular densities. Lung transplantation is sometimes performed in the setting of end-stage cystic fibrosis.

## Primary Ciliary Dyskinesia

Primary ciliary dyskinesia is an autosomal recessive disorder of abnormal motility of cilia throughout the body. These patients often have chronic sinusitis and impaired fertility, the normal functions of which are mediated by cilia. Because airway clearance is also mediated by

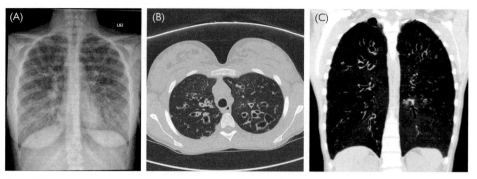

Figure 11.16 Posterior-anterior chest radiograph (**A**) and axial (**B**) and coronal (**C**) computed tomography scans in a teenager with chronic pulmonary problems show extensive bronchiectasis and bronchial wall thickening with a relative upper lobe predominance. These are classic radiographic findings of cystic fibrosis.

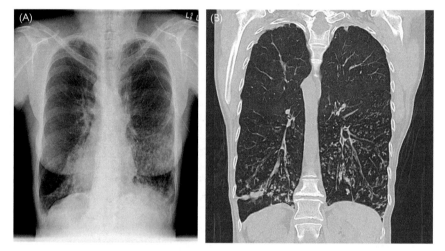

Figure 11.17 Posterior-anterior chest radiograph (**A**) and coronal chest computed tomography (**B**) in a young adult with chronic pulmonary problems and infertility show lower lobe–predominant bronchiectasis, bronchial wall thickening, scarring, and tree-in-bud opacities. These findings are similar to those of cystic fibrosis, but the basilar distribution indicates primary ciliary dyskinesia as the correct diagnosis in this case. Also note that the aortic arch and cardiac apex are on the right in the patient with situs inversus (Kartagener syndrome).

the actions of normal cilia, patients with primary ciliary dyskinesia develop airway disease, including bronchiectasis and recurrent infectious bronchiolitis.[17]

Radiographic findings are similar to those for cystic fibrosis, although the tubular bronchiectasis and air trapping tend to be more basilar predominant and milder in ciliary dyskinesia (Figure 11.17A and B) compared with the apical predominance in seen in cystic fibrosis.

**Note:** Patients with primary ciliary dyskinesia may have situs inversus because the normal left–right orientation of the organs of the chest and abdomen is initially determined by the actions of normal cilia during organogenesis. The pairing of primary ciliary dyskinesia and situs inversus is called Kartagener syndrome.

# References

1. Wiedemann JR, Saugstad AM, Barnes-Powell L, Duran K. Meconium aspiration syndrome. *Neonatal Netw.* 2008;27(2):81–87.

2. Kuhn JP, Fletcher BD, DeLemos RA. Roentgen findings in transient tachypnea of the newborn. *Radiology.* 1969;92(4):751–757.

3. Kumar A, Bhat BV. Epidemiology of respiratory distress of newborns. *Indian J Pediatr.* 1996;63(1):93–98.

4. Carey B. Neonatal air leaks: pneumothorax, pneumomediastinum, pulmonary interstitial emphysema, pneumopericardium. *Neonatal Netw.* 1999;18(8):81–84.

5. Bhandari A, Bhandari V. Pitfalls, problems, and progress in bronchopulmonary dysplasia. *Pediatrics.* 2009;123(6):1562–1573.

6. Fuloria M, Aschner JL. Persistent pulmonary hypertension of the newborn. *Semin Fetal Neonatal Med.* 2017;22(4):220–226.

7. Reuter S, Moser C, Baack M. Respiratory distress in the newborn. *Pediatr Rev.* 2014;35(10):417–428; quiz 429.

8. Epelman M, Kreiger PA, Servaes S, et al. Current imaging of prenatally diagnosed congenital lung lesions. *Semin Ultrasound CT MR.* 2010;31(2):141–157.

9. Mani H, Suarez E, Stocker JT. The morphologic spectrum of infantile lobar emphysema: a study of 33 cases. *Paediatr Respir Rev.* 2004;5(Suppl A):S313–S320.

10. Clements BS, Warner JO. Pulmonary sequestration and related congenital bronchopulmonary-vascular malformations: nomenclature and classification based on anatomical and embryological considerations. *Thorax.* 1987;42(6):401–408.

11. Lee EY, Dorkin H, Vargas SO. Congenital pulmonary malformations in pediatric patients: review and update on etiology, classification, and imaging findings. *Radiol Clin North Am.* 2011;49(5):921–948.

12. Orazi C, Inserra A, Schingo PM, et al. Pleuropulmonary blastoma, a distinctive neoplasm of childhood: report of three cases. *Pediatr Radiol.* 2007;37(4):337–344.

13. Dishop MK. Diagnostic pathology of diffuse lung disease in children. *Pediatr Allergy Immunol Pulmonol.* 2010;23(1):69–85.

14. Lucaya J, Gartner S, Garcia-Pena P, et al. Spectrum of manifestations of Swyer-James-MacLeod syndrome. *J Comput Assist Tomogr.* 1998;22(4):592–597.

15. Vichinsky EP, Styles LA, Colangelo LH, et al. Acute chest syndrome in sickle cell disease: clinical presentation and course. Cooperative Study of Sickle Cell Disease. *Blood.* 1997;89(5):1787–1792.

16. Ramsey BW. Use of lung imaging studies as outcome measures for development of new therapies in cystic fibrosis. *Proc Am Thorac Soc*2007;4(4):359–363.

17. Noone PG, Leigh MW, Sannuti A, et al. Primary ciliary dyskinesia: diagnostic and phenotypic features. *Am J Respir Crit Care Med.* 2004;169(4):459–467.

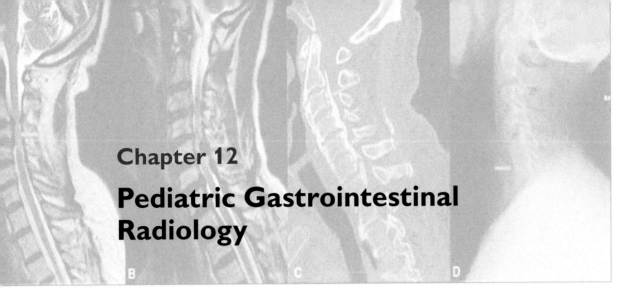

# Chapter 12

# Pediatric Gastrointestinal Radiology

*Syed Ali Raza and Anna Clebone*

**12.** Pediatric Gastrointestinal Radiology

# Neonatal High Bowel Obstruction

## Midgut Malrotation and Volvulus

The classic presentation of a neonate with midgut malrotation and volvulus (Figures 12.1 to 12.3) is bilious vomiting. The root cause of both malrotation and volvulus is an incomplete rotation of the intestines during the 10th week of gestation resulting in an abnormal or insufficient fixation of the small intestine's mesentery. In normal gestation, the intestine rotates 270 degrees counterclockwise to settle into the abdomen, with the colon at the top and sliding down the sides of the abdomen and the small bowel in the center. If this normal rotation is absent or incomplete, the bowel configuration will be abnormal, in some cases with the small intestine located to the right and the colon to the left. In malrotation, this abnormal positioning of the intestines leads to a narrowing of the mesentery and the blood supply that it carries resulting in a predisposition to intestinal ischemia.

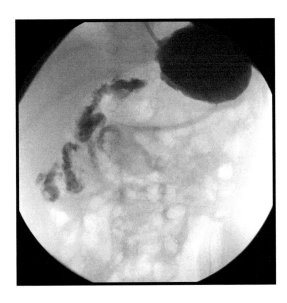

**Figure 12.1** Upper gastrointestinal series of midgut malrotation. The duodenojejunal junction is displaced downward and to the right of the spine.

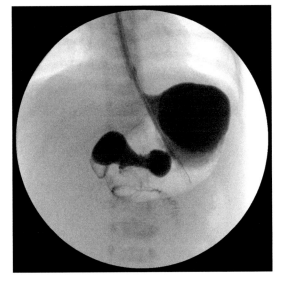

**Figure 12.2** Upper gastrointestinal series of midgut malrotation with volvulus. Seen here is a "corkscrew pattern," which shows the proximal jejunum spiraling inferiorly, with a dilated stomach and proximal duodenum.

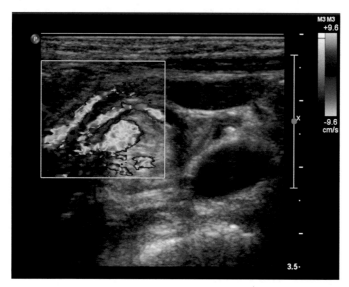

**Figure 12.3** Ultrasound of midgut malrotation with volvulus. In the *inset* is the classic whirlpool sign seen with color Doppler. Flow can be seen within the superior mesenteric vein wrapping around the superior mesenteric artery.

A volvulus occurs when, because of insufficient fixation of the mesentery, the small intestine abnormally twists around the superior mesenteric artery.[1] This is a surgical emergency. Two of the most frequently used imaging modalities are a fluoroscopic upper gastrointestinal (GI) examination with radiopaque contrast, and ultrasound, which is less sensitive and specific.[2,3]

## Duodenal Atresia

Duodenal atresia (Figure 12.4) is one of the most common causes of high intestinal obstruction in newborns and classically presents with vomiting starting at birth that is usually

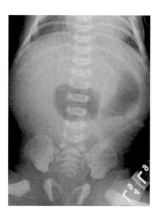

**Figure 12.4** Plain film of duodenal atresia. The characteristic double-bubble sign is seen in complete obstruction associated with duodenal atresia. The stomach and duodenum (proximal to the stenosis) are filled with air, but the rest of the abdomen is devoid of gas.

bilious (vomiting will be nonbilious in the 15% of cases in which the atresia is proximal to the ampulla of Vater). On physical exam, the infant's abdomen will often be scaphoid in appearance. It is often radiologically diagnosed with a plain abdominal radiograph, which will show the classic "double bubble" appearance, with gas only in two areas in the upper abdomen, representing the stomach and proximal duodenum. There is no need for a fluoroscopic upper GI examination because abdominal radiographs are diagnostic. Treatment is surgical repair.

**Note:** Duodenal atresia is often associated with Down syndrome.

## Duodenal Web

A duodenal web (Figure 12.5) is a congenital defect in which a membranous web (often incomplete) or intraluminal diverticulum causes obstruction in the duodenum. This can commonly be seen on a fluoroscopic upper GI examination with ingested contrast material but also can be seen on other imaging modalities such as magnetic resonance imaging (MRI).[4]

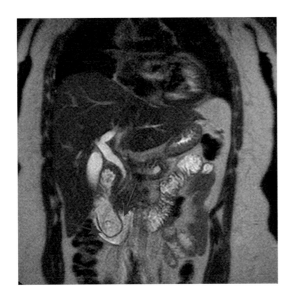

**Figure 12.5** Magnetic resonance image of a duodenal web. The classic windsock deformity is seen, in which a fluid-filled sack inside the duodenum is surrounded by a fine thin line. A similar finding may be seen on a fluoroscopic upper GI examination.

## Annular Pancreas

> **Caution!**  An annular pancreas can also cause preampullary duodenal obstruction, with a similar presentation clinically and on plain film to duodenal atresia.

Annular pancreas (Figure 12.6) is a congenital deformity caused by a defect in embryogenesis. Normally, during fetal development, two ventral pancreatic buds rotate and fuse with a single dorsal bud. If the fused ventral buds fail to rotate properly, they can encase and obstruct the duodenum, forming an annular pancreas. An annular pancreas is often asymptomatic and therefore sometimes undiagnosed until adulthood.[5] It is diagnosed with computed tomography (CT) or MRI.

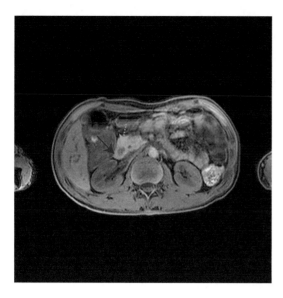

Figure 12.6 Magnetic resonance image showing pancreatic tissue (solid red arrow) encasing the second part of the duodenum (dashed green arrow).

## Pyloric Stenosis

Pyloric stenosis (Figure 12.7) is caused by an idiopathic thickening of the pyloric muscle. It classically presents with projectile nonbilious vomiting, which can in some cases distinguish it clinically from the duodenal obstruction pathologies. Pyloric stenosis presents between 1 week and 3 months of age and occurs more often in boys. Typically, these infants have a hypochloremic, hypokalemic metabolic alkalosis (although a small percentage present with hyperkalemia). It is a medical emergency to hydrate these infants and correct the electrolytes, and surgery should

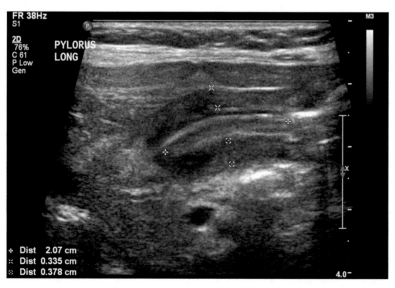

Figure 12.7 Ultrasound image showing thickening and elongation of the pylorus. The diagnosis of pyloric stenosis is often made when ultrasound measurements show a pyloric single-wall muscle thickness greater than 3 mm, a pyloric muscle length more than 15 mm, and/or a pyloric muscle diameter greater than 10 mm.

only occur after the patient is medically stabilized and normovolemic and after electrolytes approach normalization.[4] It can be diagnosed with ultrasound or fluoroscopic upper GI examination with ingested contrast material.

*Note:* Ultrasound provides less radiation and better direct visualization of the hypertrophic pylorus but is not as effective at excluding other causes of proximal obstruction as a fluoroscopic upper GI examination with ingested contrast material.

## Neonatal Low Bowel Obstruction

### Ileal Diseases

### Ileal Atresia and Meconium Ileus

Ileal atresia and meconium ileus are obstructive processes during gestation affecting the ileum. The subsequent colon becomes atrophic because of disuse, and a "microcolon" (Figure 12.8) forms in some cases.

Ileal atresia presents with bilious vomiting and abdominal distension. It is due to a fetal vascular accident in which blood flow to the ileum is compromised, and this portion of bowel becomes ischemic and narrows. On radiographs, more proximal small bowel loops are dilated because of the obstruction, but on contrast enema these loops lack contrast because the contrast is unable to move past the atretic ileum. The distal ileum, beyond the point of atresia, will therefore be small and collapsed on imaging.[4]

Meconium ileus occurs nearly exclusively in cystic fibrosis patients. Their meconium is especially thick and can accumulate in parts of the ileum, causing obstruction. Proximal dilated small bowel loops can be seen on radiographs; on contrast enema, there are multiple discrete filling defects in the ileum and colon, indicating meconium.[6] An equivalent of meconium ileus in older children with cystic fibrosis is distal intestinal obstruction syndrome, in which thick inspissated stool blocks the bowel lumen causing findings of obstruction on plain radiograph.

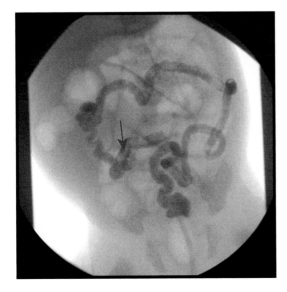

**Figure 12.8** Contrast enema displaying a "microcolon" seen in ileal disease. Note the multiple discrete, uneven filling defects (arrow) consistent with meconium ileus rather than ileal atresia.

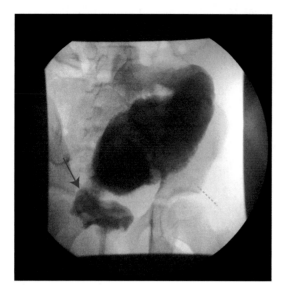

Figure 12.9 Contrast enema displaying a small-caliber rectum with mucosal contour irregularity (solid red arrow), as seen in Hirschsprung disease. More proximally, the sigmoid colon is dilated (dashed green arrow).

## Colonic Disease

### Hirschsprung Disease

Hirschsprung disease (Figure 12.9) is the result of ganglionic cells failing to migrate to parts of the distal colon or results from death of these cells after migration. The denervated segments spasm and contract, causing obstruction. The normally innervated portions more proximally become dilated. As with most low intestinal obstructive processes, plain radiograph will show multiple dilated loops of small bowel. When this is seen, further workup is done with a contrast enema rather than with an fluoroscopic upper GI examination.

### Meconium Plug Syndrome

Meconium plug syndrome (Figure 12.10) may resemble Hirschsprung disease in the distribution of obstruction in the distal colon. On contrast enema, there are multiple filling defects in the colon. An important factor for distinguishing Hirschsprung disease and meconium plug syndrome is the

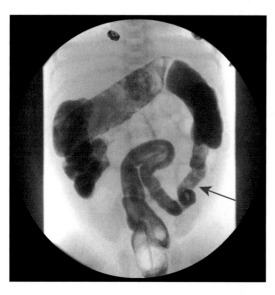

Figure 12.10 Contrast enema displaying a small left colon (arrow) with multiple filling defects. Notice that in this picture, the rectum remains larger in caliber than the sigmoid colon.

rectosigmoid ratio. In Hirschsprung disease, the rectum is often smaller than the sigmoid colon (in normal patients, the rectum is larger). In meconium plug syndrome, the rectum is "spared," and the area of abnormally small caliber involves the descending and sigmoid colon. The right and transverse colon can be dilated relative to the small left colon, which leads to it sometimes being referred to as small left colon syndrome. Both the meconium plugs and the "small left colon" typically resolve over time. A contrast enema is often both therapeutic and diagnostic in these patients.

**Note:** Unlike meconium ileus, there is no significant association with cystic fibrosis.[4]

## Bowel Obstruction Beyond the Neonatal Period

### Intussusception

Intussusception (Figures 12.11 and 12.12) is most common in children younger than 2 years of age. It occurs when a portion of bowel "telescopes" within the lumen of more distal bowel. Specifically, ileocolic intussusception involves the terminal ileum entering into the

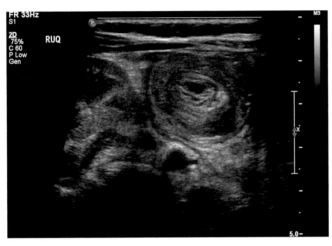

Figure 12.11 Ultrasound image of intussusception showing a mass with alternating hyperechoic and hypoechoic regions, sometimes called a "pseudo-kidney" or "doughnut sign," representing a loop of bowel within another more distal loop.

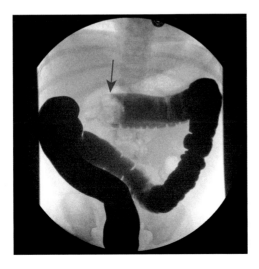

Figure 12.12 Contrast enema showing the intussusception as an intra-luminal filling defect (arrow).

colon. It can be idiopathic or can occur at a point of intestinal anatomic abnormality, called a "pathologic lead point." When idiopathic ileocolic intussusception occurs, it is often secondary to a viral illness causing lymphatic hypertrophy in the terminal ileum. Classic symptoms include abdominal pain, vomiting, and red "currant jelly" stools. When these symptoms occur, a plain radiograph or ultrasound is ordered. If either of these is suggestive of the disease, then a contrast enema is performed, which can be therapeutic in relieving the invagination of bowel.[6]

## Appendicitis versus Mesenteric Adenitis

Appendicitis (Figure 12.13) is the most common cause of pediatric bowel obstruction (after adhesions) and the number one reason for surgery in the pediatric population. It occurs when fecal matter obstructs the lumen of the appendix, and resulting inflammation, infection, and ischemia are possible.[7] This can lead to varying presentations but most commonly right lower quadrant pain and fever occur. Diagnosis is most commonly through ultrasound, CT, or MRI. Ultrasound is frequently the first line imaging modality in pediatric patients as it can be performed portably and does not subject the patient to any radiation.

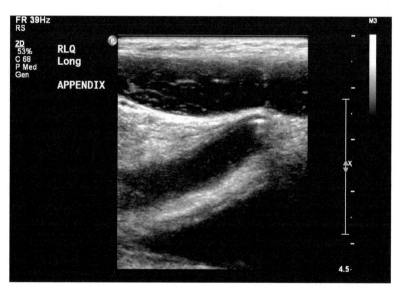

Figure 12.13 Ultrasound image of appendicitis showing an enlarged (diameter greater than 6 mm), noncompressible, fluid-filled appendix with an appendicolith at the tip.

Both CT and ultrasound can be used to diagnose mesenteric adenitis (Figure 12.14), a self-limiting inflammatory condition involving mesenteric lymph nodes. The distinction between these two disorders is important because both appendicitis and mesenteric adenitis can present with right lower quadrant pain, fevers, and vomiting. Imaging can differentiate the two by showing a normal appendix as well as prominent lymphadenopathy in the small bowel mesentery or anterior to the psoas muscle.

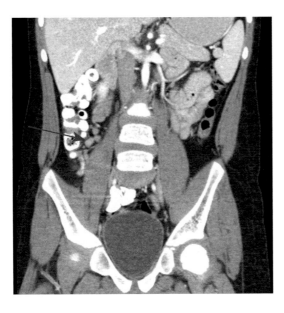

**Figure 12.14** Computed tomography scan showing a normal appendix but prominent mesenteric lymph nodes (arrow) suggestive of mesenteric adenitis.

## Enteric Duplication Cysts

Enteric duplication cysts (Figure 12.15) are congenital, lie on the wall of the bowel, and do not communicate with the lumen of the GI tract. They can grow quite large and cause bowel obstruction or a palpable mass in the abdomen.

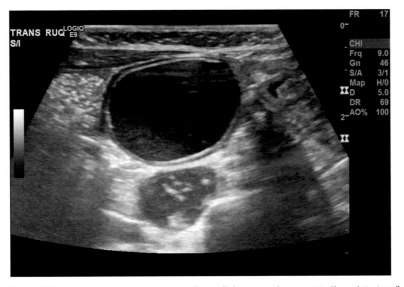

**Figure 12.15** Intra-abdominal cystic mass with a wall showing a characteristic "bowel signiture" - alternating hypoechoic (mucosal layer of bowel wall) and hyperechoic (muscular layer of bowel wall) rings. This finding indicates an eteric duplication cyst.

### Inguinal Hernia

In an inguinal hernia (Figure 12.16), a portion of bowel herniates through the abdominal wall into the inguinal region through an anatomic defect. It is more common in males and can be acquired at any point in a child's lifetime. In male patients, herniated bowel loops may extend into the scrotum. If large enough, inguinal hernia can cause bowel obstruction. A surgical emergency occurs when the piece of bowel becomes ischemic because of the hernia, resulting in incarceration or strangulation of the hernia.

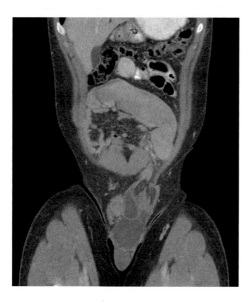

**Figure 12.16** Coronal computed tomography of the abdomen and pelvis shows fluid-filled bowel loops herniated in the left inguinal region (arrow) with surrounding fat stranding, suggesting strangulation. A dilated upstream bowel loop in the mid-abdomen indicates secondary obstruction.

## Additional Neonatal Gastrointestinal Disorders

### Necrotizing Enterocolitis

Necrotizing enterocolitis (NEC) (Figure 12.17) is a neonatal disorder in which the bowel is damaged by a combination of ischemia and infection. Bacteria entering the bowel wall can form gas

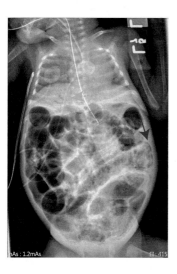

**Figure 12.17** Abdominal radiograph showing abnormal dilated tubular bowel loops throughout the abdomen in a patient with necrotizing enterocolitis. Curvilinear gas density surrounding several bowel loops (solid red arrow) represents pneumatosis intestinalis, and portal venous gas is seen as linear lucency over the liver (dashed green arrow).

bubbles that dissect into the muscularis layer of the gut and into the portal venous system. Early necrotizing enterocolitis may show fixed, dilated bowel loops on radiographs. In more advanced cases of necrotizing enterocolitis, gas can be seen in the wall of the bowel (called pneumatosis intestinalis) as well as within the portal venous system over the liver.

Necrotizing enterocolitis occurs more commonly in preterm and low-birthweight infants. Clinical signs include feeding intolerance, gastric distension, vomiting and diarrhea, lethargy, respiratory distress, hypothermia, and eventually hypotension, septic shock, and bowel perforation. Pneumoperitoneum can be seen on abdominal radiography in infants with associated bowel perforation. A large volume of air in the peritoneal space can radiographically resemble a football in that it can appear as an area in the middle of the abdomen that is hypolucent but containing the appearance of stripes from the falciform ligament.

### Meconium Peritonitis

Meconium peritonitis (Figure 12.18) occurs when the gut of the fetus perforates in utero, resulting in inflammation and aseptic peritonitis.[8] It may be caused by a wide range of intra-abdominal pathologies in the fetus. On prenatal ultrasound, it will be seen as multiple echogenic areas in the abdomen representing punctate and linear calcifications. Ascites, bowel dilation, and meconium pseudocyst may also be seen on prenatal ultrasound. On postnatal plain abdominal radiograph, calcifications can be seen in the peritoneum along with radiographic evidence of ascites. In cases with significant ascites and abdominal wall thickening, meconium peritonitis may be mistaken for hydrops.

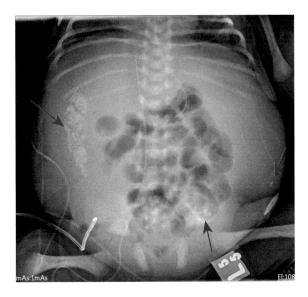

Figure 12.18 Abdominal radiograph in a newborn showing large abdominal circumference and centralization of bowel loops, indicated large-volume ascites. High-density material within the peritoneal space (arrows) represents calcified meconium in this patient with meconium peritonitis. If this radiograph were to be repeated after a short interval, the dense objects would change position because they are floating within the peritoneal space.

### Gastroschisis versus Omphalocele

See Chapter 18 "Anesthesia for Gastroschisis or Omphalocele Repair" in the companion book to this volume, titled 'Pediatric Anesthesia Procedures' published by Oxford University Press.

# Pancreas

### Cystic Fibrosis

Most patients with cystic fibrosis (Figure 12.19) develop insufficiency of the pancreas within their lifetime, which manifests as a deficient production of exocrine pancreatic enzymes. Consequences include deficiencies of fat-soluble vitamins, malnutrition, and steatorrhea. On abdominal radiographs, pancreatic calcification can sometimes be seen. In addition, on CT or MRI, intrapancreatic cysts (which may be dilated side branches), fatty replacement of the pancreas, or a dilatation of the main pancreatic duct may be seen.

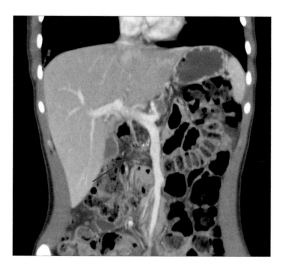

**Figure 12.19** Coronal computed tomography of the abdomen shows nearly complete fatty replacement of the pancreas (arrow) in a patient with cystic fibrosis.

### Pancreatitis

Acute pancreatitis (Figure 12.20) is an inflammatory process of the pancreas that can be due to a number of causes, including gallstones, hereditary or metabolic causes, or alcohol ingestion in teenagers. Radiographs may be normal in pancreatitis or may show dilated bowel loops related to ileus. On abdominal ultrasound in patients with pancreatitis, the pancreas can be enlarged, with

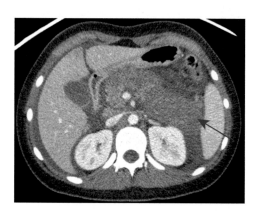

**Figure 12.20** Axial computed tomography of the upper abdomen shows an enlarged hypoattenuating pancreas (arrow) with fluid infiltration of the surrounding fat, compatible with acute pancreatitis.

heterogeneous echogenicity. CT can directly show peripancreatic fluid and edema. Complications of pancreatitis which can be seen on CT include pancreatic necrosis and fluid collections.

# Liver Tumors

### Infantile Hepatic Hemangioma

Infantile hepatic hemangioma (Figure 12.21) is a liver tumor that typically occurs in the first few months of life and is frequently seen on prenatal imaging. This benign lesion shows similar histology to hemangiomas elsewhere in the body. The lesions are frequently very large and due to their vascular nature can lead to arteriovenous shunting and high-output cardiac failure. Morbidity also occurs from consumptive coagulopathy (Kasabach-Merritt syndrome). These lesions can be characterized with MRI.

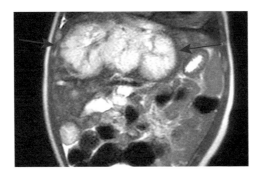

Figure 12.21 Coronal T2-weighted magnetic resonance image of the abdomen shows a large lobulated hyperintense mass in the liver (arrows) with multiple small satellite lesions, compatible with a hemangioendothelioma.

### Hepatoblastoma

Hepatoblastoma (Figure 12.22) is a highly vascular, rapidly growing solid liver tumor typically seen in children younger than 2 years of age. In newborns, hepatoblastoma is the most common

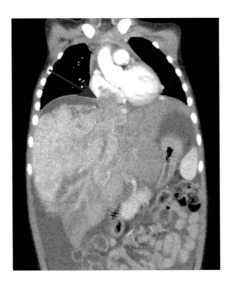

Figure 12.22 Coronal computed tomography of the abdomen shows a large infiltrating mass arising from the liver, with associated invasion of the mass into the expanded inferior vena cava and into the right atrium (arrow). This is a patient with hepatoblastoma. Note also the large-volume ascites.

malignant tumor of the liver. A hepatoblastoma may cause internal hemorrhage from rupture of the liver. Doppler studies can show the vascularity of these tumors. A spoke-wheel appearance and calcifications may be seen on CT or MRI.

## Biliary

### Biliary Cysts and Choledochal Cysts

Biliary cysts (Figure 12.23) are often congenital, and they consist of cystic dilations that can occur both intrahepatically and extrahepatically within the biliary tree (the term *choledochal cyst* refers to cysts of the extrahepatic bile duct only). Biliary cysts are uncommon and can obstruct the biliary tree and cause intrahepatic or extrahepatic dilation. A patient with jaundice or abdominal pain is often first evaluated with an abdominal ultrasound. If on ultrasound a biliary cyst is suspected, the patient usually proceeds to magnetic resonance cholangiopancreatography (MRCP), which can be used to assess for communication of the cyst with the biliary tree and the presence of associated biliary obstruction. Choledochal cysts are typically resected, in part due to a risk for malignancy.

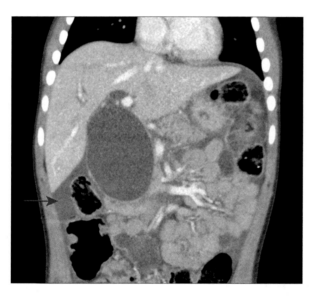

Figure 12.23 Coronal computed tomography image of the abdomen shows a large cystic mass in the area of the porta hepatis. This is a biliary fluid-filled. The gallbladder is the smaller fluid-filled structure displaced inferiorly and laterally (arrow).

### Biliary Atresia

Biliary atresia (Figure 12.24) is a neonatal extrahepatic disease in which the biliary tree is progressively obliterated and fibrosed, leading to biliary obstruction. The infant will present with jaundice in the first 2 months after birth and will require a hepatoportoenterostomy (Kasai procedure) or liver transplantation. Evaluation is with hepatobiliary scintigraphy, typically referred to as a HIDA scan. In this procedure, excretion of a radioisotope tracer from the liver to the small bowel is assessed. If excretion occurs, then the biliary tree is patent, and the diagnosis of biliary atresia is improbable. Caution must be taken, however, because in infants younger than 6 weeks, a false-negative scan may occur because the obstruction of the biliary tree may be at an early stage (and may worsen after 6 weeks of life).

### Hereditary Hemorrhagic Telangiectasia (Osler-Weber-Rendu Disease)

Hereditary hemorrhagic telangiectasia presents with bleeding from arteriovenous malformations (AVMs). These AVMs can affect the liver as well as the nasal mucosa, skin, lungs, brain, or GI

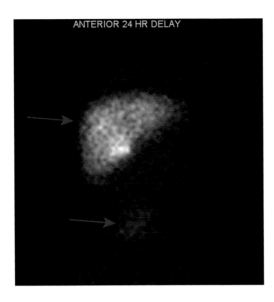

Figure 12.24 A 24-hour delayed anterior image from hepatobiliary scintigraphy (HIDA scan) shows radiotracer activity only within the liver and urinary bladder (arrows). Absence of tracer excretion into the bowel indicates biliary atresia.

tract. On CT, ultrasound, or MRI, these AVMs may appear as a large mass with a clearly defined draining vein.

## Spleen

### Polysplenia and Asplenia, Heterotaxy Syndromes

In heterotaxy syndromes, the organs of the abdomen and thorax will be variably arranged on a basis of "sidedness". For example, with classical right-sided isomerism, both lungs have a tri-lobar morphology typical of the right lung, the liver is in a transverse position, and the spleen is absent. Right isomerism is associated with severe cardiac defects. Patients with left-sided isomerism typically have two bi-lobed lungs and may present with the multiple spleens (polysplenia, Figure 12.25). Heterotaxy syndromes have a strong association with midgut malrotation.

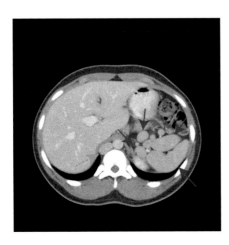

Figure 12.25 Axial computed tomography scan of the upper abdomen shows multiple round and oval soft tissue densities in the left upper quadrant (solid red arrows), representing polysplenia. This patient has a heterotaxy syndrome. Note that the inferior vena cava (dashed green arrow) is located in an abnormal position behind the diaphragmatic crura and next to the descending aorta. This is called azygous continuation of the inferior vena cava, an associated finding with heterotaxy syndrome.

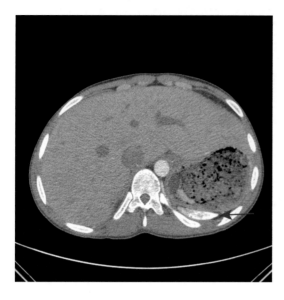

**Figure 12.26** Axial computed tomography of the upper abdomen shows a small hyperdense spleen in the left upper quadrant (arrow). In patients with sickle cell disease, the spleen autoinfarcts over time, resulting in functional asplenia.

### Sickle Cell Disease

Patients with sickle cell disease (Figure 12.26) often have effective asplenia due to progressive splenic infarction. Patients with sickle cell disease and a functioning spleen are at risk for splenic sequestration crisis, which is the pooling of red blood cells, constituting a significant percentage of total blood volume, in the spleen, with a mortality rate of up to 15%. The risk for splenic sequestration is the reason that many patients with sickle cell disease will undergo a prophylactic splenectomy even before functional asplenia can occur. In patients with sickle cell disease, the mortality rate for undergoing anesthesia was previously 1%, but careful perioperative anesthetic management, including aggressive warming techniques to ensure normothermia throughout, adequate hydration, pain management, and preoperative transfusion often to a hemoglobin of more than 10% (often performed the day before surgery), as well as close perioperative consultation with a hematologist, has decreased mortality dramatically.

## References

1. Filston HC, Kirks DR. Malrotation—the ubiquitous anomaly. *J Pediatr Surg.* 1981;16(4 Suppl 1):614–620.
2. Simpson AJ, Leonidas JC, Krasna IH, et al. Roentgen diagnosis of midgut malrotation: value of upper gastrointestinal radiographic study. *J Pediatr Surg.* 1972;7(2):243–252.
3. Pracros JP, Sann L, Genin G, et al. Ultrasound diagnosis of midgut volvulus: the "whirlpool" sign. *Pediatr Radiol.* 1992;22(1):18–20.
4. Donnelly L. *Pediatric Imaging, The Fundamentals.* Philadelphia: Saunders; 2009.
5. Sandrasegaran K, Patel A, Fogel EL, et al. Annular pancreas in adults. *AJR Am J Roentgenol* 2009;193(2):455–460.
6. Gale HI, Gee MS, Westra SJ, et al. Abdominal ultrasonography of the pediatric gastrointestinal tract. *World J Radiol.* 2016;8(7):656–667.
7. Birnbaum BA, Wilson SR. Appendicitis at the millennium. *Radiology.* 2000;215(2):337–348.
8. Uchida K, Koike Y, Matsushita K, et al. Meconium peritonitis: prenatal diagnosis of a rare entity and postnatal management. *Intractable Rare Dis Res.* 2015;4(2):93–97.

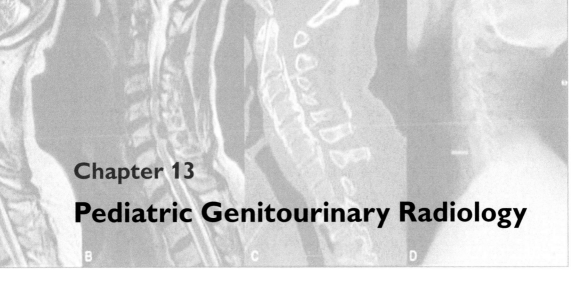

# Chapter 13

# Pediatric Genitourinary Radiology

*Mohammed Mohsin Khadir*

# Congenital

### Renal Agenesis

Renal agenesis is the congenital absence of one or both kidneys. Bilateral renal agenesis is not compatible with life, but unilateral renal agenesis generally does not affect life expectancy. In addition to being seen in several syndromes (including VACTERL), unilateral renal agenesis is associated with ipsilateral müllerian duct anomalies in girls and seminal vesicle cysts in boys[1]. Ultrasound is typically used for diagnosis. Imaging of unilateral renal agenesis demonstrates an empty renal fossa without a fusion anomaly in the remaining kidney or renal ectopia. In addition, there is usually compensatory hypertrophy of the remaining kidney (Figure 13.1).

***Pearl:*** On ultrasound, the ipsilateral adrenal gland may have a flattened morphology rather than the normal triangular shape. This is called the "lying-down adrenal" sign and is caused by the lack of normal molding by an adjacent kidney during development.

### Autosomal Recessive Polycystic Kidney Disease

Patients with autosomal recessive polycystic kidney disease (ARPKD) develop numerous very small cysts throughout both kidneys, leading to poor function. There is an association with congenital hepatic fibrosis.[2]

ARPKD is divided into four forms based on the age of presentation. The two earlier forms (perinatal and neonatal) present with severe renal disease with less extensive hepatic fibrosis. The later forms (infantile and juvenile) present with milder renal disease with severe hepatic fibrosis. The perinatal form of ARPKD has the worst prognosis with high neonatal mortality.

Prenatal or postnatal ultrasound will demonstrate enlargement of both kidneys, greater than 2 standard deviations above mean for age, with loss of the normal corticomedullary differentiation (Figure 13.2). Small renal cysts (<1 cm) are seen in about half of the patients. Large cysts are not usually seen. On magnetic resonance imaging (MRI), there is increased T2 signal throughout both enlarged kidneys.

(A)  (B)

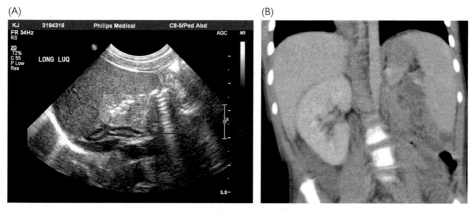

**Figure 13.1** (**A**) Ultrasound of the left renal fossa shows the "lying-down adrenal" sign, with the flat-appearing adrenal gland taking up a large portion of the renal fossa, indicating congenital absence of a normally located kidney. (**B**) Coronal computed tomography of the abdomen and pelvis demonstrates absence of the left kidney.

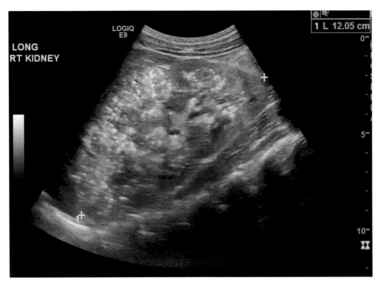

**Figure 13.2** Long view of the right kidney in a 6-year-old with polycystic kidney disease demonstrates an enlarged kidney with loss of the normal corticomedullary differentiation. There is replacement of the parenchyma with innumerable microscopic cysts, which appear echogenic owing to their small size.

## Multicystic Dysplastic Kidney
In utero, a nonfunctioning kidney is replaced by numerous cysts and dysplastic tissue. Throughout childhood, the cysts will shrink and involute. Similar to renal agenesis, unilateral disease with a normal contralateral kidney has excellent prognosis. Bilateral disease is fatal because there is no functioning renal tissue. There is a strong association with contralateral renal anomalies, particularly ureteropelvic junction obstruction.[3]

Diagnosis is typically made prenatally or in infancy. Ultrasound demonstrates a mass in the renal fossa with numerous large nonconnecting cysts of variable size (Figure 13.3) without any intervening normal renal parenchyma. The largest cysts are usually peripheral and result in a lobular contour of the kidney.

**Note:** The ultrasound appearance is important to distinguish from hydronephrosis. Hydronephrosis causes cystic-appearing dilated calyces, which connect centrally to the renal pelvis. In addition, the renal pelvis is typically the most dilated structure.

## Horseshoe Kidney and Cross-Fused Ectopia
Horseshoe kidney is the most common renal fusion anomaly. In this entity, the kidneys are fused at the lower poles across midline (Figure 13.4). Cross-fused renal ectopia presents with both kidneys fused to one side of midline. Horseshoe kidneys are asymptomatic but are more susceptible to trauma and pose a risk for hydronephrosis, renal stones, and transitional cell carcinoma. Cross-fused ectopia also poses an increased risk for hydronephrosis, renal stones, and infection.

Imaging of horseshoe kidneys demonstrates malrotated kidneys with the inferior poles of both kidneys connected by an isthmus of fibrous tissue or renal parenchyma across the midline. Imaging of cross-fused ectopia demonstrates two fused kidneys on the same side of midline, usually with a normally-located kidney fused at its lower pole to the ectopic kidney.

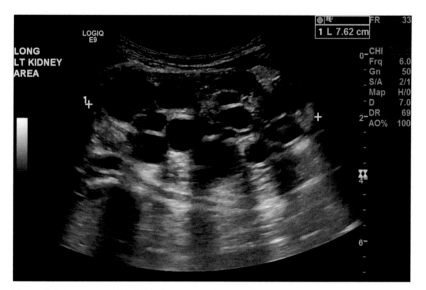

**Figure 13.3** Long view of the left kidney in a newborn with multicystic dysplastic kidney disease shows multiple large cysts replacing the left kidney. Note the absence of normal renal parenchyma.

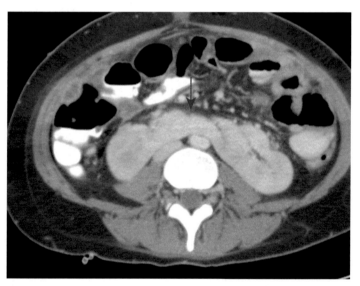

**Figure 13.4** Axial computed tomography of the abdomen in a 20-year-old with horseshoe kidney shows the right and left kidney fused at the lower poles across midline (arrow).

## Prune Belly Syndrome

Prune belly syndrome is the triad of urinary tract dilatation, bilateral cryptorchidism, and anterior abdominal wall underdevelopment.[4] The underlying etiology of the syndrome is unknown. On physical exam, patients have a large distended abdomen with redundant skin. If there is oligohydramnios, the patient may have potter facies. Prune belly syndrome occurs almost exclusively in boys. On imaging, there is severe bilateral hydroureteronephrosis with a distended urinary bladder. Scrotal ultrasound demonstrates an empty scrotum due to cryptorchidism.

## Congenital Uteropelvic Junction Obstruction

As the name implies, this is a mechanical urinary obstruction at the level of the uteropelvic junction. This can be congenital or acquired and is the most common cause of prenatal and neonatal hydronephrosis.[5] The left kidney is two times more likely to be affected than the right. Ultrasound demonstrates dilation of the renal pelvis and calyces, with normal ureters and bladder (Figure 13.5).

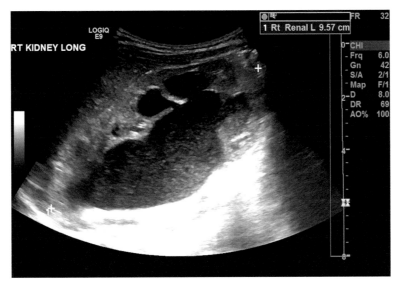

Figure 13.5 Ultrasound shows severe right hydronephrosis without ureteral dilation, compatible with ureteropelvic junction obstruction.

## Vesicoureteral Reflux

Abnormal retrograde flow of urine from the bladder into the ureters is called vesicoureteral reflux (VUR). Reflux predisposes to pyelonephritis and chronic renal parenchymal injury.

***Pearl:*** In a young child with a urinary tract infection, first suspect VUR as the etiology.[6]

VUR is most common in patients younger than 2 years and is more common in females than males. It resolves in most children as they age. VUR is graded from I to V based on its severity. Patients with a higher grade of reflux have more frequent and more severe complications of urinary tract infections (UTIs), such as renal scarring and eventually renal failure.

Diagnosis is typically made with a voiding cystourethrogram. Under fluoroscopy, contrast is instilled in the bladder. Images of the bladder and ureters are obtained at multiple angles during filling, full distension, and voiding. The exam can evaluate for the presence and grade of reflux as well as identify any anatomical abnormalities predisposing to reflux (Figure 13.6). Ultrasound can evaluate for associated hydronephrosis, scarring, or anatomic abnormalities.

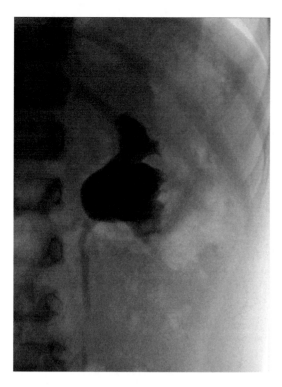

Figure 13.6 Single voiding cystourethrogram of the left kidney shows large-volume reflux from the bladder to the level of the left kidney with a dilated collecting system.

## Duplicated Collecting System

A duplicated collecting system results from incomplete fusion of the upper and lower pole renal moieties during fetal development and can present as a duplex kidney draining into either a single ureter, a bifid ureter, or two separate ureters. If there are two separate ureters, the Weigert-Meyer law applies, which states that the upper pole moiety has an ectopic ureterovesical insertion caudally and medially to the lower pole moiety ureter. Ectopic insertion of the upper pole moiety is frequently outside bladder. In males, ectopic insertion can be into the prostatic urethra. In females, ectopic insertion may be below the external urethral sphincter, which leads to incontinence.

**Note:** The upper pole ureter is often obstructed from a ureterocele, leading to dilatation of the ureter and the upper pole collecting system.

**Note:** Reflux commonly develops in the lower pole ureter.

A voiding cystourethrogram will show reflux into the lower pole ureter and contrast opacification of only the lower renal pole calyces. This classic appearance is called the "drooping lily sign."[7] Magnetic resonance (MR) urography or excretory urography can also delineate the abnormalities. There may be obstruction and dilation of the upper pole moiety and ureter (Figure 13.7). There may be scarring and atrophy of either moiety depending on the degree of obstruction or reflux. Ultrasound can delineate a duplicated collecting system but is suboptimal in evaluating the ureters.

## Ureterocele

Ureterocele is a congenital cystic dilation of the most distal aspect of the ureter. It is usually associated with ectopic insertion of the ureter into the bladder, such as with the upper pole moiety of a

(A)

(B)

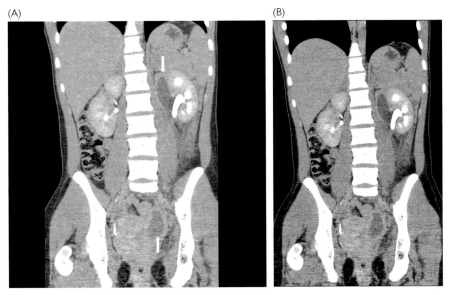

Figure 13.7 Coronal contrast-enhanced computed tomography of the abdomen and pelvis shows a duplicated left renal collecting system. Note that the upper pole of the left kidney is atrophic with a severely dilated upper pole ureter *(arrows)*. The lower pole of the kidney is normal without evidence of obstruction.

duplicated collecting system.[4] Intravesical ureteroceles herniate only into the bladder. Extravesical ureteroceles can also herniate into the bladder neck or urethra. Ultrasound demonstrates a cystic structure at the uterovesical junction (Figure 13.8A and B). A voiding cystourethrogram frequently shows a round bladder filling defect at the location of the ureterocele.

(A)

(B)

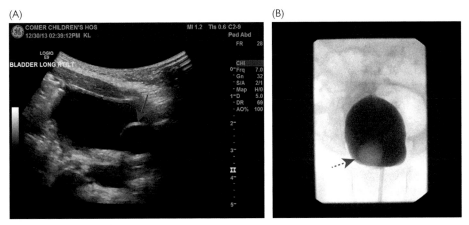

Figure 13.8 (**A**) Transverse ultrasound image of the bladder shows a cystic structure at the right vesicoureteral junction (solid arrow). (**B**) Early filling of the bladder on voiding cystourethrogram shows a round filling defect at the right vesicoureteral junction (dashed arrow) compatible with a ureterocele in this patient with a duplicated collecting system.

## Urachal Anomalies

A spectrum of congenital anomalies develop as a result of incomplete obliteration of the fetal allantoic canal, the channel between the bladder dome and the umbilicus that initially drains urine in the fetus. These urachal anomalies predispose to infection from urinary stasis and to adenocarcinoma.[8]

**Patent urachus:** The entire urachus fails to close, leading to a persistent connection between the bladder and umbilicus. These patients present with urine drainage from the umbilicus. This is the most common urachal anomaly.

**Urachal diverticulum:** The urachus remains patent only at the bladder end. Imaging demonstrates a blind-ending cystic structure (a diverticulum) at the anterior-superior aspect of the bladder (Figure 13.9).

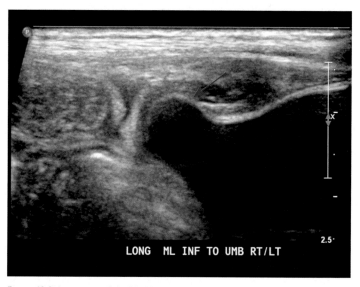

**Figure 13.9** Long view of the bladder in a 6-year-old demonstrates an outpouching at the superior aspect of the bladder (arrow), consistent with an urachal diverticulum.

**Urachal cyst:** The bladder and umbilical end of the urachus close, but a fluid-filled dilatation of the middle portion of the urachus remains. Imaging shows a midline cyst along the urachus that does not connect with the bladder or umbilicus.

**Urachal sinus:** Only the umbilical end of the urachus remains open with no communication with the bladder. These patients also present with umbilical fluid drainage.

## Bladder Exstrophy

Exstrophy describes a defect in the low midline abdominal wall with herniation of the bladder externally through the defect. Incidence is 1:10,000-50,000, and is more common in boys. Imaging demonstrates an abdominal wall defect below the umbilicus with a soft tissue mass extending through the defect from an everted bladder. Radiographs and CT show widening of the pubic symphysis more than 1 cm.

### Posterior Urethral Valves

Congenital prominence of the posterior urethral membrane leads to varying degrees of lower urinary obstruction.[4] This only occurs in males, and age of presentation depends on the severity of the obstruction. Severe obstruction will present prenatally with hydronephrosis, oligohydramnios, and pulmonary hypoplasia. Mild obstruction can present later in childhood with a poor urine stream, large postvoid residual, and abnormal voiding patterns.

Perinatal ultrasound shows a distended bladder with a thick and irregular wall. The posterior urethra will also be distended. There is typically bilateral hydronephrosis and, because of chronic obstruction, the kidneys may be dysplastic with loss of corticomedullary differentiation. A voiding cystourethrogram is the best exam for diagnosis. During voiding, a dilated posterior urethra is seen with an abrupt reduction in caliber at the level of the abnormal posterior membrane (Figure 13.10). High grade vesicoureteral reflux is also usually present.

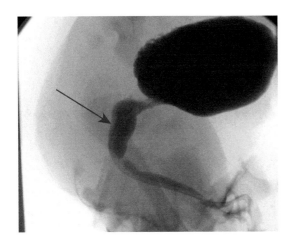

**Figure 13.10** Image from a voiding cystourethrogram in a newborn boy shows a distended and mildly trabeculated bladder with a dilated posterior urethra (arrow) compatible with a diagnosis of posterior urethral valves.

# Neuroblastoma and Wilms Tumor

### Neuroblastoma

Neuroblastoma is a malignancy arising from the primitive neural crest cells of the sympathetic system. It can arise anywhere along the sympathetic chain but is most commonly seen in the adrenal gland or the retroperitoneum.[9] In children, neuroblastoma is the third most common malignancy and the most common solid malignancy. The mean age of presentation is around 15 to 17 months, often presenting with a palpable abdominal mass.

Ultrasound is usually the first exam of choice and will demonstrate a heterogeneous adrenal mass with calcifications. CT shows an adrenal or paraspinal mass, which can cross the midline if large (Figure 13.11). Many lesions have calcification, with larger lesions demonstrating areas of necrosis and hemorrhage. Metastases to liver, bone, and lymph nodes are common. MRI shows a large heterogeneous mass with variable and heterogeneous enhancement.

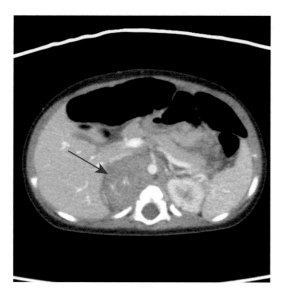

Figure 13.11 Axial contrast-enhanced computed tomography scan of an infant shows a soft tissue mass O(arrow) arising from the right adrenal gland. Note that the mass contains calcifications and encases local vasculature. This is neuroblastoma.

## Wilms Tumor

Wilms tumor is a malignant pediatric renal tumor arising from primitive metanephric blastema. It is associated with multiple syndromes, most notably Beckwith-Wiedemann syndrome and WAGR syndrome (Wilms tumor, aniridia, genitourinary abnormalities, and intellectual disability).[10] Wilms tumor is the most common pediatric renal mass. The typical age of presentation is 3 to 4 years with a palpable abdominal mass.

Ultrasound is usually the first exam of choice and shows a large heterogeneous mass arising from the kidney. CT and MRI also show a large heterogeneous mass arising from the kidney; normal renal tissue can be seen partially wrapping around tumor at its margin, creating a "claw sign" (Figure 13.12). A minority of lesions have calcifications.

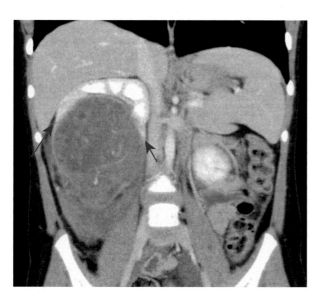

Figure 13.12 Coronal contrast-enhanced computed tomography scan of a 6-year-old shows a large heterogeneous mass arising from the right kidney. Note the "claw sign" (arrows) as normal renal tissue wraps around the margin of the tumor.

*Pearl:* Distinguishing Wilms tumor and neuroblastoma on imaging is important. Wilms tumor arises from the kidney, as opposed to neuroblastoma, which typically arises from the adrenal gland. Also, Wilms tumor rarely contains calcifications, which are commonly seen in neuroblastoma. Additionally, Wilms tumor tends to displace adjacent vascular structures, as opposed to neuroblastoma, which encases them.

## Reproductive

### Ovarian Torsion

> **WARNING!!** Ovarian torsion is an emergency requiring surgical detorsion.

Twisting of the vascular pedicle supplying the ovary and fallopian tube causes venous obstruction and can eventually lead to infarction of the ovary. Torsion can be intermittent or sustained.[11] Presentation is usually acute with severe unilateral pelvic or lower abdominal pain, nausea, and vomiting.

Ultrasound is the first exam of choice. It will show an enlarged ovary with follicles displaced to the periphery of the ovary and the ovary displaced to midline (Figure 13.13A and B). Color Doppler findings in the ovary are variable, from completely absent venous flow to normal flow, due to a dual blood supply from both the ovarian and uterine arteries. Most patients have free pelvic fluid. MRI demonstrates similar findings to ultrasound and may also directly demonstrate the twisted vascular pedicle, which is pathognomonic for ovarian torsion.

*Pearl:* Ovarian enlargement is the strongest predictor of torsion.

(A)        (B)

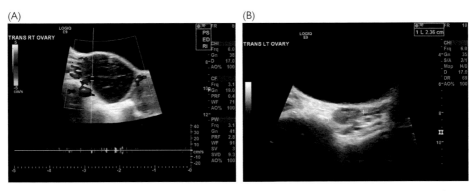

Figure 13.13 (**A**) Pelvic ultrasound image of a 15-year-old girl with pain shows an enlarged hypoechoic right ovary with peripheral follicles and abnormal blood flow. (**B**) The normal left ovary is shown for comparison.

### Testicular Torsion

> **WARNING!!** Testicular torsion is an emergency requiring surgical detorsion and orchiopexy.

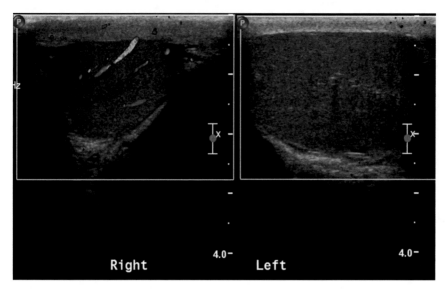

Figure 13.14 Sagittal color Doppler ultrasound of both testicles in a 14-year-old shows a mildly enlarged left testicle with absent blood flow, compatible with testicular torsion.

Twisting of the testis and spermatic cord results in occlusion of the vascular supply to the testis. Torsion can eventually lead to infarction of the testis. Patients present with acute scrotal pain. Pain may be intermittent if spontaneous detorsion occurs.

Ultrasound is the first exam of choice. Comparison should be made with the contralateral normal testis. The torsed testis is enlarged and heterogenous compared with the normal testis (Figure 13.14). Twisting of the spermatic cord may be seen. Depending of the degree of torsion, decrease or complete absence of blood flow to the testis can be seen on color Doppler images.[12,13] Prophylactic contralateral orchiopexy is also performed.

### Epididymo-orchitis

Epididymo-orchitis refers to inflammation of the epididymis or the epididymis and testis. Orchitis alone is rare and classically seen in patients with mumps. Epididymo-orchitis usually presents with a more gradual onset of pain, swelling, and erythema of scrotum. Patients can be febrile. Elevation of the scrotum relieves pain.[13]

*Note:* Scrotal elevation does not relieve pain in testicular torsion.

Ultrasound is the modality of choice. Comparison should be made with the contralateral normal testis. The effected epididymis is enlarged and heterogenous with increased blood flow to both the epididymis and testis on color Doppler images (Figure 13.15). Reactive hydrocele and scrotal wall thickening are common.

*Note:* Blood flow may be decreased or completely absent with testicular torsion.

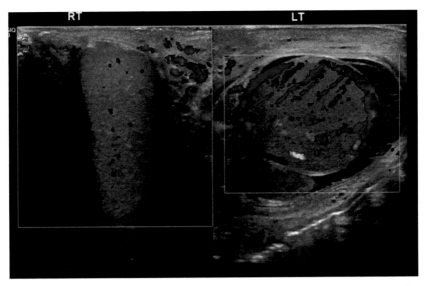

Figure 13.15 Comparison color Doppler image of both testicles shows that the left testicle is enlarged and markedly hyperemic compared with the right.

## Hydrocele

Hydrocele is a serous fluid collection between the layers of the tunica vaginalis. Fluid surrounds the testis and spermatic cord. Hydrocele presents as painless scrotal enlargement and may be congenital or acquired. Acquired etiologies include epididymitis, surgery, tumor, and trauma.[12] Ultrasound is the modality of choice and will demonstrate fluid surrounding the testis without internal blood flow (Figure 13.16). Fluid may be simple-appearing or can have septations or debris.

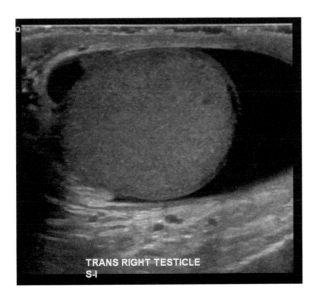

TRANS RIGHT TESTICLE
S-I

Figure 13.16 Ultrasound image of the right testicle demonstrates fluid surrounding the right testicle, consistent with a simple hydrocele.

## Varicocele

Varicocele is characterized by dilated veins in the pampiniform plexus due to retrograde flow in gonadal vein. Varicocele is the most common mass in the spermatic cord. Patients present with scrotal swelling and pain. Varicocele is typically left-sided and less commonly bilateral.

> **Caution!** An isolated right varicocele should raise concern for an intra-abdominal mass compressing the draining gonadal vein.

Ultrasound is the exam of choice. The veins of the pampiniform plexus will be serpiginous and measure greater than 2 to 3 mm. During Valsalva, the veins increase in size and there can be reversal of flow[12] (Figure 13.17A and B).

(A)                                                (B)

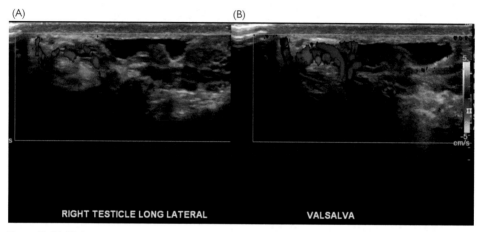

RIGHT TESTICLE LONG LATERAL                VALSALVA

Figure 13.17  (**A**) Lateral color Doppler ultrasound images of the right testicle show dilated pampiniform veins with little blood flow. (**B**) During Valsalva maneuver, the blood flow markedly increases in the veins.

## Testicular Tumors

Primary testicular tumors consist of germ cell tumors, making up two-thirds of cases, and non–germ cell tumors. Germ cell tumors include yolk sac tumor, teratoma, embryonal carcinoma, choriocarcinoma, mixed germ cell tumor, and seminoma. Seminoma is the most common testicular germ cell tumor (Figure 13.18). Non–germ cell tumors include Leydig cell tumors, Sertoli cell tumors, and juvenile granulosa cell tumors.[14]

Lymphoma can also involve the testis. Presentation is typically a painless testicular mass. Embryonal rhabdomyosarcoma is a classic extratesticular scrotal tumor in a child. Imaging characteristics are nonspecific for testicular tumors. Lesions can have cystic areas, calcifications, and variable echogenicity on ultrasound. Surgical pathology is needed for definitive diagnosis.

## Sacrococcygeal Teratoma

Sacrococcygeal teratoma is a germ cell tumor arising from the pluripotential cells of the notochord at the sacrum-coccyx level. It is the most common congenital tumor in the fetus and neonate and is more commonly seen in girls. Sacrococcygeal teratoma is typically diagnosed prenatally and can be benign or malignant.

***Pearl:*** Surgical resection includes removal of the coccyx bone, which decreases recurrence rate.

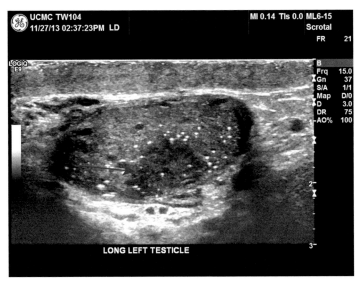

Figure 13.18 Ultrasound image of the left testicle shows a hypoechoic mass (arrow) on a background of testicular microlithiasis. Orchiectomy was performed, and pathology showed a seminoma.

Like teratomas elsewhere in the body, this tumor may be comprised of all three germ layers and can contain teeth, hair, fat, and other material. MRI is frequently performed for characterization of sacrococcygeal teratoma. Imaging demonstrates a large heterogeneous mass with solid and cystic components arising from the coccyx (Figure 13.19).[15] The mass can contain calcifications, fat, solid soft tissue, and cystic components.

**Note:** The mass can grow internally into the presacral area and externally into the buttock. Prognosis is best in patients with tumors extending predominantly externally and is worst in patients with entirely intrapelvic tumors.

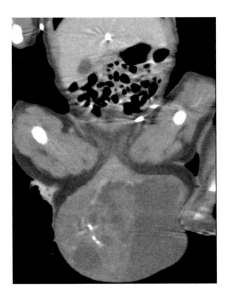

Figure 13.19 Coronal contrast-enhanced computed tomography scan of a newborn shows a large heterogeneous exophytic pelvic mass. The mass contains cystic and fatty components as well as calcifications. Findings are compatible with a sacrococcygeal teratoma.

# References

1. Li S, Qayyum A, Coakley FV, Hricak H. Association of renal agenesis and mullerian duct anomalies. *J Comput Assist Tomogr.* 2000;24(6):829–834.
2. Turkbey B, Ocak I, Daryanani K, et al. Autosomal recessive polycystic kidney disease and congenital hepatic fibrosis (ARPKD/CHF). *Pediatr Radiol.* 2009;39(2):100–111.
3. Atiyeh B, Husmann D, Baum M. Contralateral renal abnormalities in multicystic-dysplastic kidney disease. *J Pediatr.* 1992;121(1):65–67.
4. Berrocal T, Lopez-Pereira P, Arjonilla A, Gutierrez J. Anomalies of the distal ureter, bladder, and urethra in children: embryologic, radiologic, and pathologic features. *Radiographics.* 2002;22(5):1139–1164.
5. Kleiner B, Callen PW, Filly RA. Sonographic analysis of the fetus with ureteropelvic junction obstruction. *AJR Am J Roentgenol.* 1987;148(2):359–363.
6. Stein R, Dogan HS, Hoebeke P, et al. Urinary tract infections in children: EAU/ESPU guidelines. *Eur Urol.* 2015;67(3):546–558.
7. Callahan MJ. The drooping lily sign. *Radiology.* 2001;219(1):226–228.
8. Parada Villavicencio C, Adam SZ, Nikolaidis P, et al. Imaging of the urachus: anomalies, complications, and mimics. *Radiographics.* 2016;36(7):2049–2063.
9. Woodward PJ, Sohaey R, Kennedy A, Koeller KK. From the archives of the AFIP. *Radiographics.* 2005;25(1):215–242.
10. Lowe LH, Isuani BH, Heller RM, et al. Pediatric renal masses: Wilms tumor and beyond. *Radiographics.* 2000;20(6):1585–1603.
11. Chang HC, Bhatt S, Dogra VS. Pearls and pitfalls in diagnosis of ovarian torsion. *Radiographics.* 2008;28(5):1355–1368.
12. Aso C, Enríquez G, Fité M, et al. Gray-scale and color Doppler sonography of scrotal disorders in children: an update. *Radiographics.* 2005;25(5):1197–1214.
13. Avery LL, Scheinfeld MH. Imaging of penile and scrotal emergencies. *Radiographics.* 2013;33(3):721–740.
14. Coursey Moreno C, Small WC, Camacho JC, et al. Testicular tumors: what radiologists need to know—differential diagnosis, staging, and management. *Radiographics.* 2015;35(2):400–415.
15. Kocaoglu M, Frush DP. Pediatric presacral masses. *Radiographics.* 2006;26(3):833–857.

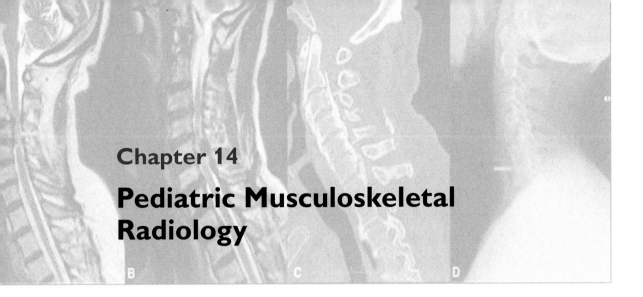

# Chapter 14

# Pediatric Musculoskeletal Radiology

*Nicholas Florence*

# Trauma

Long bones in growing children contain cartilaginous growth plates, epiphyses, and a thick, strong periosteum. The immature skeleton is more malleable than adult bone, and bones are more likely to bend with force than to break or splinter.[1] Fracture patterns are important to orthopedists, and the relative positioning of the major fragments determines potential surgical management. Fractures are simple if there are two fragments and comminuted if there are more than two (Figure 14.1). The term *compound* is used if the overlying skin is broken.

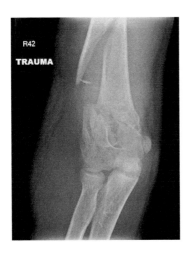

Figure 14.1 Elbow radiograph in a child after trauma shows a complex comminuted fracture of the distal humerus with displacement and angulation of the primary distal fragment. The prognosis is worse for these types of fractures.

## Buckle Fractures

Also called "torus fractures," buckle fractures occur with compressive loading. They are incomplete impaction fractures around all or part of the circumferential cortex of metaphyseal bone, where the bone is most porous (Figure 14.2). They most commonly occur in preschool-aged children.[1] A classic scenario is a distal radial buckle fracture resulting from a fall on an outstretched hand.

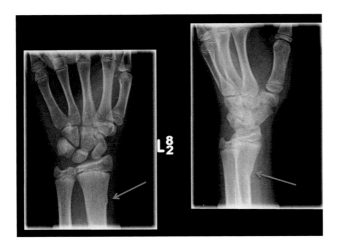

Figure 14.2 Left wrist radiographs in a child with trauma show a buckle fracture of the distal radius (arrows).

## Bowing and Greenstick Fractures

Bowing can occur with angular force on bone. Angulation beyond the bone's capacity of bowing results in a greenstick fracture, which only extends through part of a bone's width (Figure 14.3).[1,2]

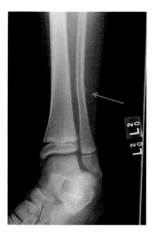

Figure 14.3 Ankle radiograph shows an incomplete oblique lucency of the distal fibular diaphysis (arrow) consistent with a greenstick fracture.

## Growth Plate (Physis) Fractures

Some of the most clinically important fractures in children are those involving the growth plate (or physis) because of their potential to disturb bone growth and development, often leading to considerable morbidity.[3] The Salter-Harris classification system describes common patterns of physeal fractures. Salter-Harris fractures are classified from 1 to 5, with a higher classification indicating a poorer prognosis (Figure 14.4A–E).[2,3]

**Note:** Prognosis is primarily dependent on the degree of arterial disruption.[3]

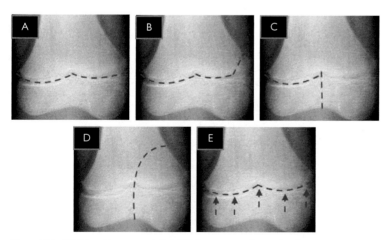

Figure 14.4 (**A**) Salter-Harris type 1 (6–8.5%) fractures result in isolated transection through the physis, without involvement of the epiphysis or metaphysis.(**B**) Type 2 is the most common Salter-Harris fracture (73–75%). It extends through the physis and a corner segment of the metaphysis, sparing the epiphyseal ossification center and resulting in the metaphyseal "corner sign." (**C**) Type 3 (6.5–8%) fractures involve an oblique or vertical cleavage line through the epiphysis extending to and horizontally through the physis to the periphery, and sparing the metaphysis. (**D**) Type 4 (10–12%) fractures split vertically through the epiphysis, physis, and metaphysis. (**E**) Salter-Harris type 5 fractures are rare axial crush injuries with physial destruction. There are often no acute radiographic findings, but follow-up imaging will likely show growth arrest at the affected physis. (From Rogers LF, Poznanski AK. Imaging of epiphyseal injuries. *Radiology*. 1994;191(2):297–308. doi:10.1148/radiology.191.2.8153295.)

***Pearl:*** Radiographs are the initial diagnostic study of choice in Salter-Harris injuries, with computed tomography (CT) reserved for characterization of known fractures and for surgical planning.

## Stress Fractures

> **Caution!** Stress fractures may also mimic benign or malignant bone lesions on radiographs but usually have more subtle periosteal reactions (Figure 14.5A).

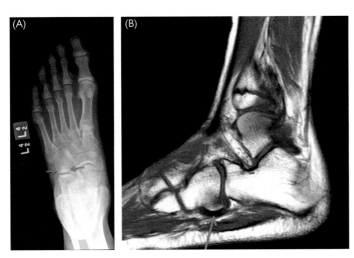

**Figures 14.5** Images from an 11-year-old girl with ankle pain and swelling. (**A**) Foot radiograph shows a poorly defined sclerotic area in the cuboid (arrow 1) compatible with a stress fracture. (B) Magnetic resonance imaging shows low T1 signal along the lateral aspect of the base of the cuboid (arrow 2). No discrete fracture line is present.

A stress fracture is mechanical failure of a bone that occurs over time as a result of repetitive, additive stresses applied to the bone. Risk factors include any repetitive activity that is new, different, or rigorous (such as distance running).[4] Plain radiographs are the initial study of choice but are often normal, especially early after the fracture.[5]

Magnetic resonance imaging (MRI) is more sensitive and specific in demonstration of associated pathophysiologic changes, which are often dark (low signal) on T1-weighted imaging (Figure 14.5B) and bright (high signal) on T2-weighted imaging. Radionuclide bone scanning has been considered the gold standard of evaluating stress fractures because subtle change in bone metabolism may be present weeks before radiographic findings. The classic finding is focal fusiform cortical uptake of technetium-99m (Figure 14.6).[4]

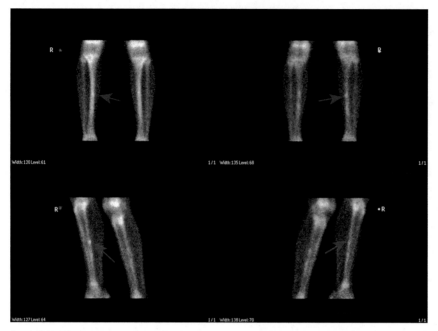

Figure 14.6 Three-phase nuclear medicine bone scan shows increased uptake of radiotracer technetium-99m MDP in the right tibial diaphysis on delayed imaging (arrows), consistent with an acute stress fracture.

## Elbow

Knowledge of the normal elbow anatomy is critical to diagnosing subtle pediatric fractures. A line drawn through the anterior cortex of the humerus on a true lateral view should pass through the anterior third of the capitellum. A line drawn through the proximal radial shaft should intersect the capitellum on every projection (Figure 14.7).[2] There are extracapsular fat pads of the anterior and posterior elbow that are of diagnostic utility in trauma radiographs.

***Pearl:*** If the fat pads are abnormally prominent, there is a mildly elevated chance of an associated elbow fracture.

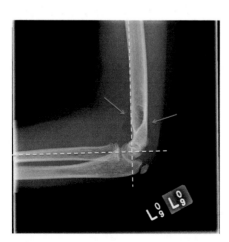

Figure 14.7 Lateral elbow radiograph of an 8-year-old after trauma. Although no fracture line is seen, an elevated anterior fat pad and a visible posterior fat pad (the "fat pad sign") are suggestive of an occult elbow fracture, usually a supracondylar fracture in this age group. The radiocapitellar and anterior humeral lines are in appropriate position.

Supracondylar fractures are the most common elbow fractures in children and usually occur with falls. The fracture line extends transversely through the coronoid and olecranon fossae. There is frequently posterior displacement of the distal fragment, so the anterior humeral line passes anterior to the capitellum (Figure 14.8). [1]

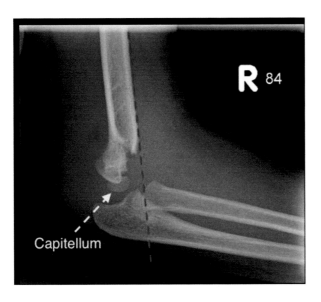

Capitellum

**Figure 14.8** Elbow radiograph of a 3-year-old with pain and deformity after a fall on an outstretched hand. There is a transverse fracture of the supracondylar humerus with posterior angulation of the distal fragment, causing the anterior humeral line to pass anterior to the capitellum.

A medial epicondylar ossification center appears at about 5 years of age and fuses during the middle teenage years.[1] Avulsion fractures of the medial epicondyle (Figure 14.9) are common.

***Pearl:*** Medial epicondyle injury, also known as "little league elbow" often occurs in young pitchers from repetitive overhand throwing, which applies valgus stress on a vulnerable elbow without fused growth plates.

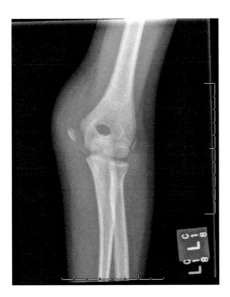

**Figure 14.9** Elbow radiograph of a 9-year-old shows an avulsion injury of the medial humeral epicondyle.

*Pearl:* Subluxation of the radial head relative to the capitellum (with a disrupted radiocapitellar line) is called "nursemaid's elbow" and results from pulling a young child's forearm with the hand and wrist in pronation. Supination of a slightly flexed elbow will reduce this subluxation and result in a normal-appearing radiograph.

## Avulsion Injuries of the Pelvis and Hip

Pelvic fractures in children do not typically disrupt the pelvic ring unless there is severe trauma. Avulsion fractures are far more common. The most common avulsion fractures are of the ischial tuberosity where the hamstring muscles attach (Figure 14.10) and of the iliac spines at the origin of the sartorius or rectus femoris tendon. They frequently occur in athletic adolescents.[2]

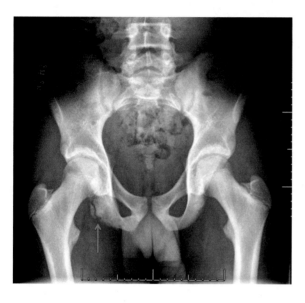

**Figure 14.10** Pelvis radiograph of a 16-year-old shows a healing avulsion fracture of the right ischial tuberosity.

### Knee

Osgood-Schlatter disease is an injury of the proximal tibia at the attachment of the patellar tendon and is thought to be due to repetitive microtrauma (Figure 14.11A and B). This typically occurs in young athletes who participate in sports that involve jumping, such as basketball. Soft tissue swelling and fragmentation of the tibial tuberosity and, uncommonly, there will be an avulsion fracture of the tibial tuberosity.[6]

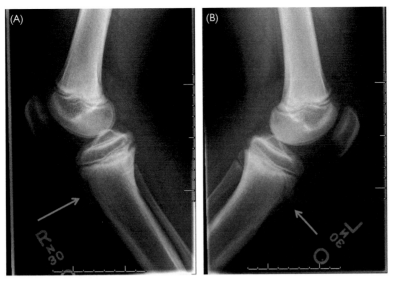

Figure 14.11 Knee radiographs in an adolescent with 2 months of pain showing bilateral patellar tendon thickening at the site of insertion at the tibial tuberosity and fragmentation of the tibial tubercle. These findings are compatible with Osgood-Schlatter disease.

**Note:** Symptoms invariably resolve following fusion of the growth plate.

Sinding-Larsen-Johansson disease is an incomplete avulsion injury of the inferior pole of the patella caused by repetitive tensile force exerted by the infrapatellar tendon (Figure 14.12). This has a similar pathophysiology to Osgood-Schlatter disease.[6]

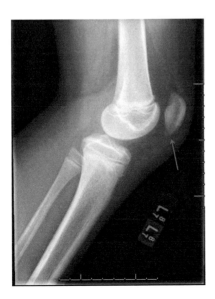

Figure 14.12 Knee radiograph of a 12-year-old with pain showing fragmentation of the inferior pole of the patella, compatible with Sinding-Larsen-Johansson disease.

## Nonaccidental Trauma

Nonaccidental trauma (child abuse) is vitally important to recognize on imaging. There may be several injuries of different ages or an injury that is unexplained by the given history or is more extensive or severe than the history would suggest.[1] For example, a tibial fracture in a child too young to walk should raise suspicion of child abuse.

High-suspicion injuries are those with a low probability of accidental occurrence based on the typical activities of children. A specific fracture that is pathognomonic for child abuse is a metaphyseal corner or "bucket handle" fracture (Figure 14.13A and B). This injury can only occur from forces of violent back and forth shaking of a young child. Other high-suspicion fractures are posterior and lateral rib fractures, often at multiple contiguous levels.[2,3]

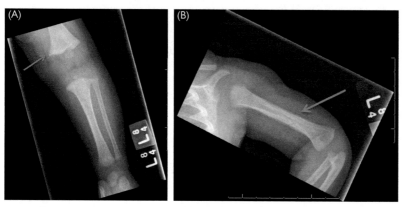

Figure 14.13 (A) Left lower leg radiograph and (B) left arm radiograph in a 4 month old. The image of the lower extremity shows cortical irregularity of the medial aspect of the distal femoral metaphysis indicating a corner fracture. The image of the arm shows a nondisplaced spiral fracture with periosteal reaction indicating healing changes. These findings are highly suspicious for nonaccidental trauma.

The most common nonaccidental fractures are spiral fractures of the femur and tibia, fractures of the clavicle, and fractures of the skull, particularly of the occiput.[1] Skeletal survey is the recommended screening modality to evaluate for evidence of child abuse.

**Pearl:** Central nervous system injury is the major source of morbidity and mortality related to nonaccidental pediatric trauma.[2]

## Mimics of Child Abuse

Rickets may cause widespread bowing deformities and stress fractures and must be kept in the differential diagnosis when considering child abuse. Osteogenesis imperfecta is a congenital abnormality of collagen synthesis that results in fragile bones susceptible to fracturing. Wormian bodies are small intrasutural bones in the skull that can occur in association with genetic conditions such as osteogenesis imperfecta and may mimic skull fractures from child abuse.[2] Toddler's fractures, named because of their high incidence in newly ambulatory children, are spiral or oblique fractures that are isolated to a single tibial diaphysis from torsion at the level of the foot (Figure 14.14).[2] They must be distinguished from injuries of a battered child.

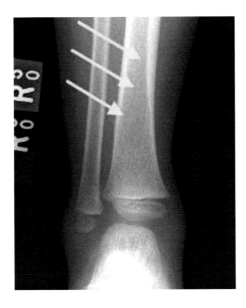

Figure 14.14 Right leg radiograph in a 2-year-old with pain. A spiral lucency through the distal diaphysis of the right tibia is consistent with a toddler's fracture.

## Infection and Inflammation

### Osteomyelitis

Infection of the bone is usually secondary to hematogenous spread in children who present with acute febrile systemic illness.[1]

**Note:** The epiphysis is usually initially spared because the metaphyseal arteries do not cross the growth plate. In neonates, the metaphyseal arteries penetrate the growth plate, so there may be early epiphyseal involvement and growth plate destruction.[7]

> **WARNING!!** Plain radiographs are insensitive and nonspecific for osteomyelitis. They typically appear normal until about 5 to 7 days into the course.

On radiographs, a nidus of infection will be lytic, sometimes expansile, and may have associated periostitis or surrounding sclerosis.[2]

In very young children or infants, bone scintigraphy is often helpful in showing multifocal increased uptake (Figure 14.15A).[2] However, MRI is the modality of choice in suspected osteomyelitis in older children, adolescents, and adults. MRI will show low T1 signal and high T2 signal within the bone.[7] Enhancement will be variable with nonenhancing or rim-enhancing abscesses and enhancing vascularized inflammatory tissue (Figure 14.15B). Brodie abscesses, often seen in young children and infants, represent subacute osteomyelitis with intraosseous abscess formation (Figure 14.15B).[1]

**14.** Pediatric Musculoskeletal Radiology

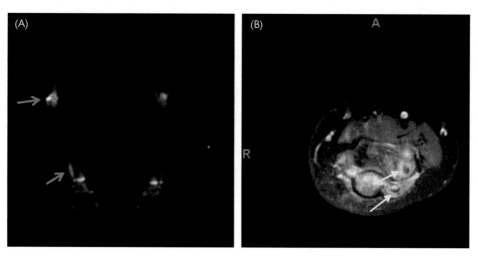

**Figures 14.15** Images of an eleven-year-old male with fever, elbow pain and decreased range of motion. (**A**) Nuclear medicine bone scan bone-scan shows increased uptake at the left elbow and distal ulna, suggesting acute inflammation. (**B**) Post-contrast T1-weighted MRI shows ring-enhancing lesions in the distal left humerus and proximal left ulna/radius. These findings are compatible with osteomyelitis.

## Septic Arthritis

Septic arthritis is a surgical emergency that is more common in children. It will present clinically as a painful, swollen joint and/or a limp in a sick, febrile child.[2]

*Pearl:* If there is suspicion for septic arthritis, an utrasound examination should be obtained to evaluate for a joint effusion (Figure 14.16). Although presence of an effusion is nonspecific, its absence rules out septic arthritis because this is an early sign. This is followed by frank destruction of the cartilage.[7] Treatment is often started empirically. However, only cytology or microbiology of aspirated fluid is truly diagnostic.

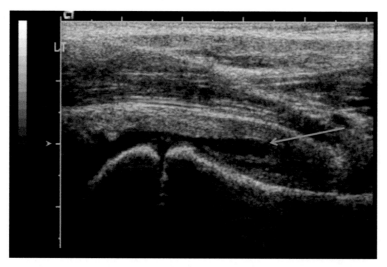

**Figure 14.16** Hip sonogram shows fluid in the left hip joint synovial space (arrow) and surrounding soft tissue thickening, compatible with a joint effusion from either transient synovitis or septic arthritis.

## Transient Synovitis

Transient synovitis is an aseptic inflammatory reaction of the hip, probably of postviral etiology. It is the most common cause of hip pain or limp in children younger than 10 years. As in septic arthritis, an effusion will be present on ultrasound. However, children with transient synovitis are generally well appearing and often have a history of recent respiratory tract infection. Transient synovitis is self-limited.[8]

## Juvenile Idiopathic Arthritis

Juvenile idiopathic arthritis is a clinical diagnosis with a frequently shifting classification system. It presents with synovitis in multiple joints. Radiographs will appear normal early in the disease, and later findings may include enlarged epiphyses, periostitis, accelerated bone maturation, or osteoporosis. Unlike adult inflammatory arthritis, joint erosions are not typically seen. Advanced disease commonly leads to growth disturbances.[2]

# Congenital and Developmental

### Developmental Dysplasia of the Hip

Developmental hip dysplasia is often a result of femoroacetabular disarticulation in utero, more commonly occurring in girls. Abnormal newborn hip positioning is related to oligohydramnios or breech orientation. There is subsequent underdevelopment of the femoral head and the acetabulum.

***Pearl:*** Although a "clunking" hip may make the diagnosis clinically, ultrasound is the initial imaging modality of choice in the neonatal period and will demonstrate less than 50% coverage of the femoral head by the acetabulum and an angle of less than 60 degrees between the ilium and the acetabular roof (Figure 14.17A and B).[9]

(A)                                             (B)

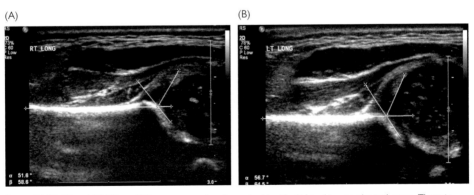

**Figure 14.17** (**A** and **B**) Bilateral hip sonograms in a 1-week-old with clicking hips on physical exam. There is less than 50% coverage of the femoral head and alpha angles of less than 60 degrees bilaterally. These findings are compatible with bilateral hip dysplasia.

### Slipped Capital Femoral Epiphysis

Slipped capital femoral epiphysis is a Salter-Harris type 1 fracture of the open femoral head growth plate with radiographs showing posterior and medial displacement of the femoral head

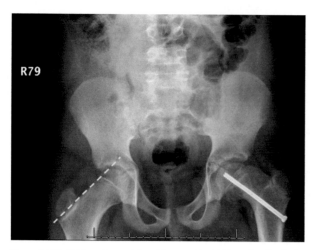

**Figure 14.18** Pelvis radiograph in a 12-year-old with 2 weeks of right hip pain. Both femoral necks are laterally displaced with respect to the femoral heads. This patient has bilateral slipped capital femoral epiphyses. The left side has already been pinned.

relative to the femoral neck (Figure 14.18). It is most commonly seen in obese adolescent males. Hip dysplasia, early arthritis, and avascular necrosis are potential complications.[1] Treatment is orthopedic pinning through the physis to prevent further slippage.

***Pearl:*** MRI is more sensitive than radiographs, showing abnormally increased T2 signal around the growth plate, even early in the disease process when alignment across the growth plate may be normal. [7]

## Legg-Calvé-Perthes Disease

Legg-Calvé-Perthes disease is idiopathic avascular necrosis of the femoral head. It is usually seen in school-aged children. Pelvic radiographs may show flattening or fragmentation of the femoral head epiphysis with subchondral fractures and joint space widening due to overgrowth of the articular cartilage (Figure 14.19). MRI may reveal earlier findings such as edema and loss of T1 bone marrow signal.[1]

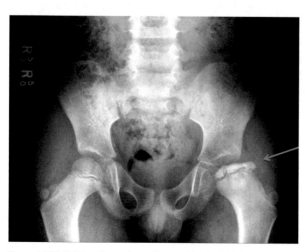

**Figure 14.19** Pelvis radiograph in a 9-year-old girl with left hip pain showing flattening of the left femoral epiphysis with sclerosis and fragmentation. This is consistent with avascular necrosis of the left hip, also known as Legg-Calvé-Perthes disease.

## Blount Disease

Blount disease, or tibia vara, is a developmental injury of the medial aspect of the proximal tibial growth plate. Lateral growth progresses normally, leading to a varus deformity and beaking of the medial metaphysis on radiographs (Figure 14.20).[2]

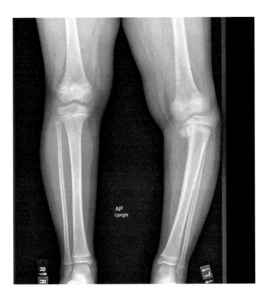

Figure 14.20 Lower extremity radiograph showing varus deviation of the left tibia with narrowing of the medial tibiofemoral compartment in this 9-year-old girl, compatible with Blount disease.

## Congenital Foot Deformities

Talipes equinovarus, or clubfoot, includes varus angulation of the hindfoot and medial deviation with inversion of the forefoot, usually from a combination of genetic and intrauterine factors. These deformities are often mild and infrequently require surgical correction, which may involve surgical release of soft tissues and realignment of the foot.[1]

Tarsal coalition is abnormal bony, fibrous, or cartilaginous bridging between two tarsal bones, most commonly between the talus and calcaneus. This occurs bilaterally in up to 50% of cases and can result in flat rigid feet.[7]

***Pearl:*** CT and MRI are both helpful in demonstrating the anatomy of coalition. Radiographs may show secondary signs such as talar beaking (spurring of the anterior superior talus) and dorsal subluxation of the navicular.

A host of other abnormalities in the hindfoot, midfoot, and forefoot may lead to flatfoot deformity, also known as "pes planus." This entity is best demonstrated on lateral radiographs as decreased calcaneal pitch.

## Scoliosis

Scoliosis is lateral curvature of the spine greater than 10 degrees in the coronal plane. It occurs more commonly in females and is usually idiopathic. Other etiologies include growth asymmetry, neoplastic or infectious damage, trauma, and asymmetric neuromuscular control of the spine.[7] Scoliosis is best evaluated with radiographs covering the entire spine to document the magnitude and extent of curvature (Figure 14.21).

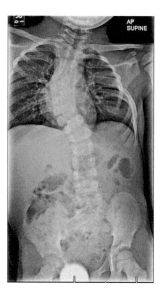

Figure 14.21  Spine radiograph showing dextroscoliosis with multiple vertebral and rib anomalies in a 5-year-old boy. This is a case of congenital scoliosis.

## Neurofibromatosis

Musculoskeletal manifestations of neurofibromatosis include scoliosis (sometimes severe), focal abnormal bone formation (e.g., sphenoid wing dysplasia), posterior vertebral body scalloping, rib thinning, long bone bowing, and pseudoarthroses (Figure 14.22).[2]

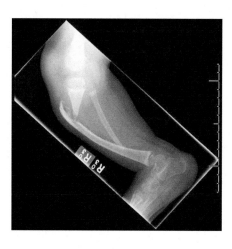

Figure 14.22  Leg radiograph of a 4-year-old boy with neurofibromatosis showing severe fracture deformity and pseudoarthrosis of the proximal right tibia, a characteristic skeletal manifestation of neurofibromatosis.

## Osteogenesis Imperfecta

Osteogenesis imperfecta is a congenital disorder of abnormal collagen synthesis resulting in thin, osteoporotic, and fragile bones (Figure 14.23A and B). There is a spectrum of severity, with radiographic findings ranging from the adult-onset osteoporosis to scattered childhood fractures to prenatal death.[1]

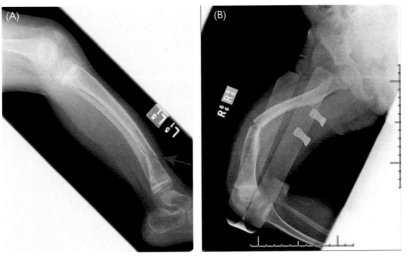

Figure 14.23 Radiographs of a 3-year-old girl showing (**A**) a spiral fracture of left tibia (arrow) and, 1 month later, (**B**) a transverse fracture of the right femur. Multiple pathologic fractures of thin osteoporotic bone are compatible with this patient's history of osteogenesis imperfecta.

## Osteopetrosis

Osteopetrosis is a rare hereditary disorder of osteoclast activity resulting in reduced bone resorption and incomplete or absent bone remodeling. Radiographs can demonstrate dense bones (universal osteosclerosis) without medullary cavities (Figure 14.24), broadened metaphyses (the so-called Erlenmeyer flask deformity), bowing of long bones, and bone-within-a-bone appearance of flat or small bones. Transverse pathologic fractures are a frequent occurrence.[1]

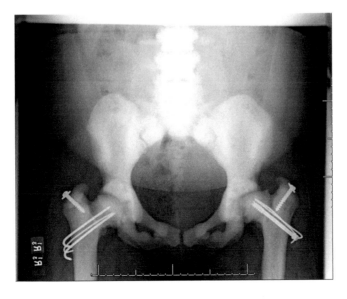

Figure 14.24 Pelvis radiograph of a 15-year-old boy status post–bilateral hip fixations. The medullary spaces are obliterated with diffuse sclerosis consistent with osteopetrosis.

## Dwarfism

Dwarfism is the condition of disproportionately shortened stature. The most common type of dwarfism is achondroplasia, which is a genetic defect of endochondral ossification resulting in generalized shortening of bones formed in this manner. The most striking radiographic feature is shortening of the limbs and phalanges (Figure 14.25) with progressive disproportionate macrocephaly because ossification of the calvarium is unaffected.[1]

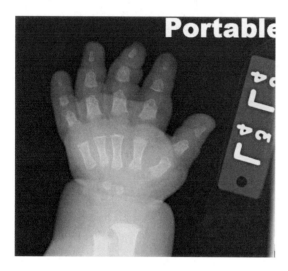

Figure 14.25 Hand radiograph of a 6-month-old shows short, widened metacarpals and phalanges, compatible with achondroplasia.

# Metabolic

### Rickets

Rickets is a disorder of bone mineralization and cartilage formation at the growth plates in skeletally immature children. It primarily results from vitamin D deficiency predominantly from dietary, malabsorptive, or metabolic reasons or from inadequate exposure to ultraviolet radiation. There are associated low serum concentrations of calcium and phosphorus. Radiographs show widening of the physes, fraying and cupping of the metaphyses, bowing of long bones (Figure 14.26), osteoporosis, and fractures.[7]

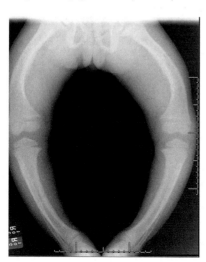

Figure 14.26 Lower extremity radiograph of a 5-year-old boy with a history of rickets. There is marked bowing of the bilateral femurs, tibiae, and fibulae as well as metaphyseal cupping and fraying.

> **Caution!** "Looser zones," transverse lucencies in long bones representing demineralized osteoid, are another characteristic feature of rickets and are often mistaken for fractures.[6]

**Note:** The "rachitic rosary" is a sign characterized by cupping and widening of anterior ribs at the costochondral junctions.[2]

## Scurvy
Scurvy is a rare disorder of cartilage production and maintenance due to vitamin C deficiency and can be seen in young children.[7]

**Note:** A classic sign is the Wimberger sign, a large central lucency within the epiphysis.[7] There may also be hemarthrosis and subperiosteal hemorrhage with elevation of the periosteum.[1]

## Lead Poisoning
Lead poisoning can result from ingestion of lead found in paint chips, toys, and food stored in lead containers. It can also result from inhalational exposure. Calcium is replaced with lead in growing bone, particularly in the metaphyses of the femur and tibia. Transverse dense lines can be seen adjacent to the physes on radiographs (Figure 14.27A and B).[1]

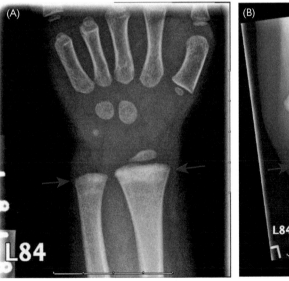
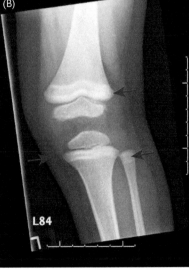

Figure 14.27 (**A** and **B**) Radiographs of a 2-year old boy show transversely oriented sclerotic bands at the metaphyses of the left radius, ulna, femur, tibia, and fibula (arrows). This is consistent with lead poisoning in the setting of elevated serum lead levels.

## Gaucher Disease

Gaucher disease is a lipid storage disorder caused by a genetic deficiency of glucocerebrosidase and subsequent overabundance of glucocerebrosides. Classically seen are Erlenmeyer flask–shaped long bones, osteopenia, medullary expansion, cortical thinning, and avascular necrosis of the femoral head, usually bilaterally.[7]

## Mucopolysaccharidoses

Mucopolysaccharidoses are a group of lysosomal storage diseases characterized by the inability to metabolize and subsequent buildup of mucopolysaccharides. Radiographs demonstrate variable degrees of dysostosis multiplex, a syndrome of complex skeletal abnormalities involving nearly any of the bones of the body.[1]

# Neoplastic and Other Aggressive Lesions

Important radiologic factors of bone lesions include location within the skeleton and within the involved bone, features of the lesion, aggressiveness and growth rate of the lesion, and age and gender of the patient.

## Osteosarcoma

Osteosarcoma is the most common primary malignancy of bone. These tumors comprise osteoid-producing cells and are most common in patients younger than 30 years. There are many subtypes; conventional intramedullary-based osteosarcomas typically occur at the metaphysis. Approximately 50% occur around the knee, either at the distal femur or proximal tibia. They can be painful or may be discovered as the result of a pathologic fracture, a common sequela of any bone tumor.[10]

The appearance of osteosarcomas on imaging is that of variable mixes of lytic (lucent) and blastic (dense) components (Figure 14.28).[5] The lytic areas represent the noncalcified portions of the tumor. Interspersed blastic foci represent mineralized osteoid matrix.

***Pearl:*** Cortical penetration often occurs rapidly, which can result either in a Codman triangle, where only the raised edge of the periosteum is ossified, or a perpendicular "sunburst" periosteal reaction.[1]

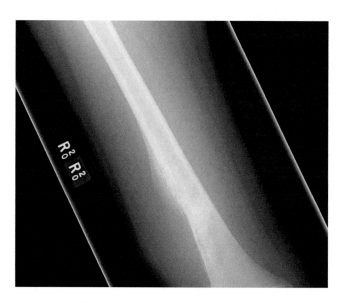

**Figure 14.28** Femur radiograph of an eleven-year-old with gradual onset of pain shows sclerosis and extensive lamellated periosteal elevation in the distal femoral metadiaphysis, compatible with osteosarcoma.

## Ewing Sarcoma

Ewing sarcoma belongs to a group of tumors called small cell sarcomas and is likely neuroectodermal in lineage.[11] Seventy-five percent occur before the age of 20 years. This is the most common primary bone tumor in children younger than 10 years.[1] Typical locations include the femur, tibia, fibula, humerus, scapula, sacrum, and pelvis. They are classically found in the metadiaphysis, particularly in the femur, and begin in the intramedullary space with a "permeative" lytic or mixed lytic and sclerotic appearance (Figure 14.29A and B).[7] With progression, they penetrate the cortex, resulting in the classic "onion-skinning" of the periosteum on radiographs. Finally, they invade the surrounding soft tissue, which is well demonstrated on CT and MRI.

***Pearl:*** A soft tissue mass associated with Ewing sarcoma is often larger than one associated with osteosarcoma.

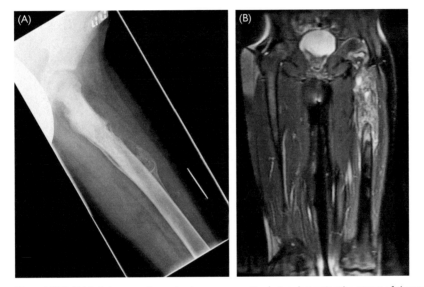

Figure 14.29 (**A**) Left femur radiographs show a permeative lesion destroying the cortex of the proximal femur. (**B**) Coronal MR image shows a large associated soft tissue mass. This was a Ewing sarcoma.

## Osteoid Osteoma

Osteoid osteomas are benign but painful bone-forming neoplasms. They begin as a small, central, and relatively radiolucent nidus made up of osteoid and fibrovascular tissue with surrounding reactive sclerosis (Figure 14.30A and B). They are usually cortically based. Sometimes the nidus may be obscured by peripheral sclerosis, and CT or MRI may be required to illustrate its presence.[5]

***Pearl:*** Osteoid osteomas may be treated with surgical resection or CT-guided radiofrequency ablation.[5]

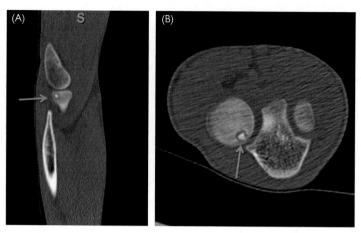

Figure 14.30 (**A** and **B**) Elbow computed tomography images of a 14-year-old with gradual onset of right elbow pain shows a small sclerotic nidus surrounded by a lucent ring in the right radial head (arrows). This is compatible with a benign osteoid osteoma.

## Eosinophilic Granuloma

Eosinophilic granulomas are common benign pediatric bone lesions and are twice as common in boys as in girls. They are the typical skeletal lesions of Langerhans cell histiocytosis. The tumors are usually solitary and are composed of a mix of inflammatory cells, including macrophages and (rarely) eosinophils. They involve flat bones (most commonly the skull), vertebrae, or metadiaphysis of long bones.[12]

On radiographs, they can appear as expansile lytic lesions with well-defined borders and sclerotic remodeling later in their course. They can be permeative and aggressive (Figure 14.31) and, in some cases, may even breach the cortex, inciting a periosteal reaction or involving the overlying soft tissues.[1,12]

*Pearl:* In the skull, the lucencies have a beveled appearance due to differing involvement of the inner and outer tables.[12]

## Osteochondroma

Osteochondromas are benign abnormal outgrowths of surface cartilage that produce bone as they expand outward, resulting in normal bone matrix with a cartilage cap. They are very common in adolescents, typically appearing as bony protuberances near the growth plates.

*Pearl:* A disorder called multiple hereditary exostoses presents with several osteochondromas and an increased risk for sarcomatous degeneration.

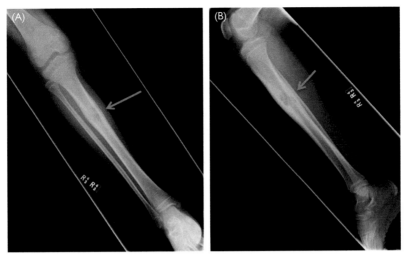

Figure 14.31 Right leg radiographs of a child with pain show a lucent lesion with extensive surrounding sclerosis and cortical thickening, compatible with an eosinophilic granuloma.

## Enchondroma

> **Caution!** Chondrosarcomas, in contrast, are typically larger, occur in older patients, penetrate past the cortex, and have a more permeative "moth-eaten" appearance.

Enchondromas are common benign radiolucent neoplasms of young adulthood occurring within the intramedullary cavity, typically at the metaphyses.[13] They are small (<3 cm) expansile lesions, often thinning the cortex without penetrating it. They can contain foci of calcification. They are most commonly encountered in the hands, femur, and humerus in patients older than 10 years.[7]

Enchondromatoses are sporadic nonhereditary conditions, such as Ollier disease, in which numerous enchondromas are seen (Figure 14.32). They are associated with an increased risk for chondrosarcoma later in life.[2]

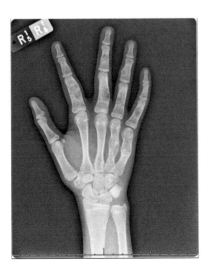

Figure 14.32 Hand radiograph in a 14-year-old girl shows multiple enchondromas of the metacarpals and phalanges, consistent with Ollier disease.

## Nonossifying Fibromas and Fibrous Cortical Defects

Nonossifying fibromas are very common non-neoplastic lesions in which bone is replaced by benign fibrous tissue. They affect patients from 4 years of age to adolescence. They are considered "do not touch" lesions because of their benign course and classic imaging appearance. They are eccentric lytic lesions with well-defined sclerotic borders that cause scalloping of the surrounding bone, sometimes described as having a "bubbly" appearance. Fibrous cortical defects occur within the cortex and are smaller than nonossifying fibromas, which occur within the medullary cavity. They occur most commonly in the metaphysis and can occasionally lead to pathologic fractures.[5]

## Fibrous Dysplasia

> **Caution!**   There is a propensity for fibrous dysplasia to mimic other more aggressive lesions on radiography.

Fibrous dysplasia is a benign non-neoplastic disorder of fibroblasts that lay down fibrous tissue containing dysplastic trabeculae of immature bone. The lesions have a classic hazy or "ground-glass," appearance (Figure 14.33). Most lesions are monostotic (involving only one bone), and polyostotic lesions may be associated with syndromes, including McCune-Albright syndrome. Fibrous dysplasia can predispose to bowing deformities and pathologic fractures.[1,14]

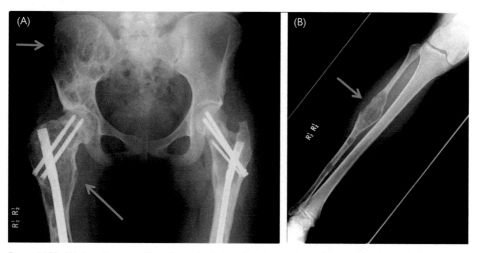

**Figure 14.33** (A) Anterior-posterior radiograph of the pelvis shows a lucent lesion within the neck and intertrochanteric and subtrochanteric regions of the right femur with a ground-glass matrix, compatible with fibrous dysplasia. (B) Anterior-posterior radiograph of the right leg shows similar lesions in the fibula.

## Aneurysmal Bone Cysts

Aneurysmal bone cysts are lucent cystic lesions of bone that expand and "balloon out" the surrounding bone. They consist of fibrovascular tissue with cystic spaces filled with blood and serosanguinous fluid, leading to the characteristic fluid-fluid levels seen on CT or MRI (Figure 14.34A—D).[5]

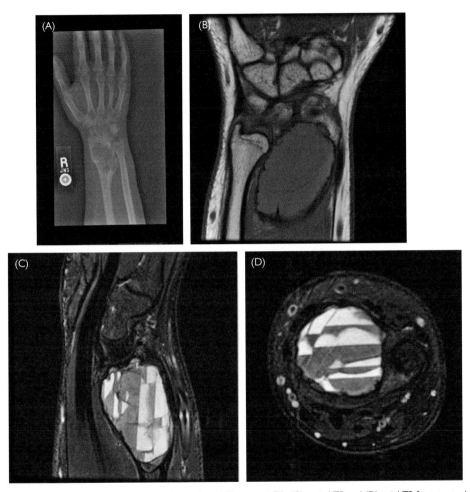

**Figure 14.34** (A) Posterior-anterior radiograph and (B) coronal T1, (C) sagital T2 and (D) axial T2 fat saturated magnetic resonance images of the right wrist of a 20-year-old woman with arm pain. Radiographs show a lucent intramedullary lesion with periosteal elevation as well as a soft tissue component with lateral swelling. Magnetic resonance imaging shows a bone lesion with cortical penetration, periosteal elevation, and multiple cystic chambers with fluid-fluid levels. These findings are compatible with an aneurysmal bone cyst.

## Unicameral (Simple) Bone Cyst

Unicameral bone cysts are round lesions filled with serous or serosanguinous fluid and therefore have fluid attenuation levels on CT.

**Pearl:** A helpful specific sign on radiographs is a fractured bone fragment that has fallen dependently within the lesion, indicating that the lesion is fluid filled.[5]

# References

1. Chew FS. *Skeletal Radiology: The Bare Bones*. 3rd ed. Philadelphia: Wolters Kluwer/ Lippincott Williams & Wilkins; 2010.
2. Mandell J. *Core Radiology: A Visual Approach to Diagnostic Imaging*. Cambridge, UK: Cambridge University Press; 2013:3.
3. Rogers LF, Poznanski AK. Imaging of epiphyseal injuries. *Radiology*. 1994;191(2):297–308. doi:10.1148/radiology.191.2.8153295.
4. Anderson MW, Greenspan A. Stress fractures. *Radiology*. 1996;199(1):1–12. doi:10.1148/ radiology.199.1.8633129.
5. Brant WE, Helms CA. *Fundamentals of Diagnostic Radiology*. 4th ed. Philadelphia: Wolters Kluwer Health/Lippincott Williams & Wilkins; 2012.
6. Greenspan A. *Orthopedic Imaging: A Practical Approach*. Philadelphia: Lippincott Williams & Wilkins; 2004.
7. Yochum TR, Rowe LJ. *Yochum and Rowes Essentials of Skeletal Radiology*. Philadelphia: Lippincott/Williams & Wilkins; 2005.
8. Miralles M, Gonzalez G, Pulpeiro JR, et al. Sonography of the painful hip in children: 500 consecutive cases. *AJR Am J Roentgenol*. 1989;152(3):579–582.
9. Õmeroğlu H. Use of ultrasonography in developmental dysplasia of the hip. *J Child Orthop*. 2014;8(2):105–113. doi:10.1007/s11832-014-0561-8. doi:10.1148/ radiographics.17.5.9308111.
10. Murphey MD, Robbin MR, Mcrae GA, et al. The many faces of osteosarcoma. *Radiographics*. 1997;17(5):1205–1231.
11. Maygarden SJ, Askin FB, Siegal GP, et al. Ewing sarcoma of bone in infants and toddlers: a clnicopathologic report from the Intergroup Ewing's Study. *Cancer*. 1993;71(6):2109–2118. doi:10.1002/1097-0142(19930315)71:6<2109::aid-cncr2820710628>3.0.co;2-1.
12. David R, Oria RA, Kumar R, et al. Radiologic features of eosinophilic granuloma of bone. *AJR Am J Roentgenol*. 1989;153(5):1021–1026. doi:10.2214/ajr.153.5.1021.
13. Manaster B. Incidental enchondromas of the knee. *Yearbook Diagnostic Radiol*. 2009;2009:79. doi:10.1016/s0098-1672(08)79265-8.
14. Fitzpatrick KA, Taljanovic MS, Speer DP, et al. Imaging findings of fibrous dysplasia with histopathologic and intraoperative correlation. *AJR Am J Roentgenol*. 2004;182(6):1389–1398. doi:10.2214/ajr.182.6.1821389.

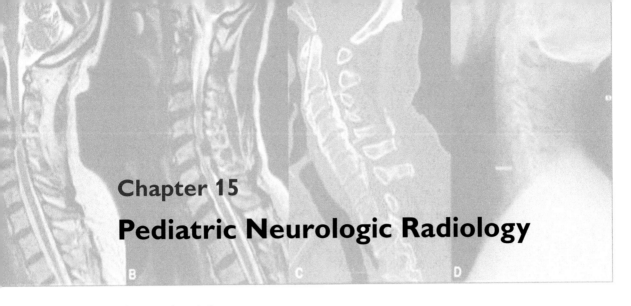

# Chapter 15
# Pediatric Neurologic Radiology

*Christopher Johnson*

# Head and Neck

## Choanal Atresia and Congenital Piriform Aperture Stenosis

Both choanal atresia and congenital piriform aperture stenosis are congenital abnormalities that may restrict or obstruct airflow through the nasal passage and nasopharynx. Each has a spectrum of severity that directly corresponds to time of diagnosis and severity of symptoms, most significantly seen as respiratory distress in the newborn. Most cases require surgical treatment.[1,2]

**Note:** These abnormalities may lead to difficulty with nasogastric tube placement or securing a nasal airway.

Choanal atresia is the most common congenital abnormality involving the nasal cavity. It can be categorized as bony (minority) or mixed bony and membranous (majority). Computed tomography (CT) is the diagnostic tool of choice. Bony subtype findings include bony narrowing through the maxilla or pterygoid plate (Figure 15.1). Membranous subtype findings include soft tissue narrowing in the posterior nasal passage as it enters the nasopharynx.

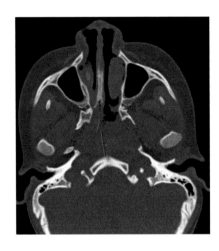

Figure 15.1  Axial computed tomography with narrowing of the right posterior nasal passage from bony elements (arrow). Comparison can be made to the normal left nasal passage.

Piriform aperture stenosis is similarly diagnosed with CT. It is differentiated by the narrowing occurring in the anterior nasal cavity as it enters the nasal passage (Figure 15.2). Findings included medial deviation of the maxilla, which narrows the passage.

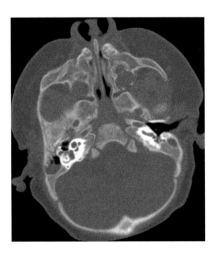

Figure 15.2  Axial computed tomography showing bilateral narrowing of the anterior nasal passages as the maxilla deviates medially.

**Pearl:** An additional common diagnostic clue is the presence of a single midline incisor, or megaincisor (Figure 15.3).

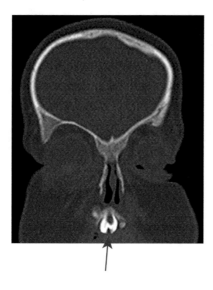

Figure 15.3 Coronal computed tomography of a pediatric patient with a single, bicuspid midline incisor (arrow).

### Branchial Cleft Cysts

Branchial cleft cysts are benign cystic masses that form as a remnant of the cervical sinus of His during development. Although frequently present at birth, they may not be diagnosed until they become enlarged or secondarily infected. Branchial cleft cysts can vary greatly in size as well as location. The most common derivative (second branchial cleft cyst) will arise in the lateral neck near the angle of the mandible to the low anterior neck, typically just anterior to the sternoclei-domastoid muscle (Figure 15.4). Symptomatic patients require complete surgical resection for treatment.[3,4]

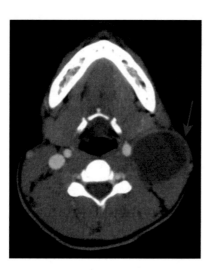

Figure 15.4 Axial computed tomography demonstrating a simple, rounded fluid collection in the lateral left neck (arrow).

Branchial cleft cysts are most easily diagnosed with CT or magnetic resonance imaging (MRI). Findings show a simple cystic structure in the anterior neck lateral to the midline. Using the anterior margin of the sternocleidomastoid as a reference point can help lead to the diagnosis.

**Note:** While branchial cleft cysts should not typically enhance with contrast, they may show enhancement in the setting of superimposed infection.

### Thyroglossal Duct Cyst

Thyroglossal duct cysts are benign cystic masses that form as a remnant of the embryologic thyroglossal duct. The thyroglossal duct runs along the midline of the neck from the base of the tongue to the level of the thyroid gland. These cysts can arise anywhere along this pathway. Similar to branchial cleft cysts, these often present as an asymptomatic mass or may have superimposed infection. Curative treatment is through surgical resection.[3,4]

**Pearl:** Recurrence rates are lowest when resection includes removal of the middle portion of the hyoid bone, called a Sistrunk procedure.

Thyroglossal duct cysts are easily diagnosed with ultrasound, CT, or MRI. Findings show a cystic structure in the anterior neck at the midline, most commonly at the level of the hyoid (Figure 15.5).

**Note:** Thyroglossal duct cysts should not typically enhance with contrast, but they may show enhancement in the setting of superimposed infection.

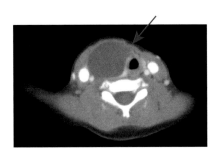

**Figure 15.5** Axial computed tomography showing a rounded simple fluid collection in the anterior neck (arrow). Although it appears to deviate to the right, a small beak can be seen anterior to the trachea at its origin.

### Fibromatosis Colli

Fibromatosis colli is a benign entity marked by enlargement of the sternocleidomastoid muscle. The process is non-neoplastic, although it may mimic a neck mass. It is seen soon after delivery. Although the etiology is unclear, it may be related to birth trauma because it has an increased incidence in breech or forceps deliveries. Treatment is conservative, typically with physical therapy or stretching exercises.

Ultrasound is the diagnostic tool of choice. Findings demonstrate a smooth, ovoid area of thickening within the sternocleidomastoid muscle. It has variable echogenicity but should appear similar to the surrounding muscle (Figure 15.6). Comparison to the contralateral normal side is useful for diagnostic confirmation.[3]

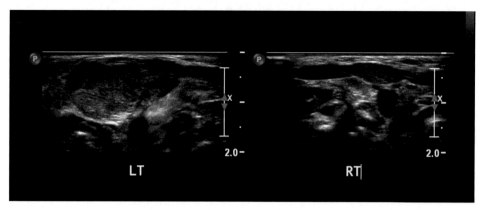

Figure 15.6 Transverse ultrasound images of the left sternocleidomastoid muscle with ovoid area of thickening and no distinct mass. Comparison can be made to the normal right side.

## Retinoblastoma

Retinoblastoma is a malignancy of the retina typically seen early in childhood. It classically results in a loss of the normal red reflex from a camera flash, called leukocoria. While it can be isolated as a unilateral mass, it is not uncommon to present bilaterally, particularly in the setting of heritable variants. Although benign entities occur in the globe, retinoblastoma is the most common intraocular tumor in children. A localized tumor can be treated with enucleation/surgical resection.

CT and MRI are most useful in diagnosis. CT findings include an amorphous intraocular mass arising from the posterior aspect of the globe in the region of the retina (Figure 15.7). The characteristic finding is calcification within the mass, which helps to differentiate it from other intraocular pathology.[5]

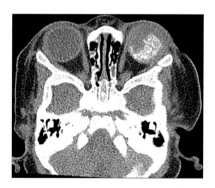

Figure 15.7 Axial computed tomography showing a heavily calcified mass filling the left globe lining the surface of the retina. Comparison can be made to the normal right eye.

# Spine

## Tethered Cord

Tethered cord syndrome is traditionally diagnosed clinically with imaging used for confirmation. Because the caudal aspect of the cord is affected, involving the conus and filum terminale,

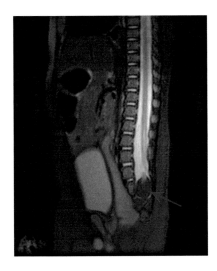

**Figure 15.8** Sagittal magnetic resonance image of the spine showing the spinal cord extending caudally to the level of the sacrum. A round low signal mass (arrow) indicates a lipoma as the etiology for the tethered cord.

symptoms relate to lumbosacral levels. Classically, these include lower extremity sensorimotor issues and bladder dysfunction.

Diagnosis is best made on sagittal MRI, although ultrasound can be used in newborns. The conus normally terminates at the L1–2 level. In patients with a tethered cord, the filum is thickened and adherent (tethered) to a lipoma or fibrolipoma at the terminal aspect of the spine (Figure 15.8). The tethering also stretches and thins the cord, resulting in a low-lying conus below the level of L2. Additional findings can include spinal dysraphism, fusion anomalies, or abnormal vertebral segmentation.[3,6]

## Spinal Dysraphism

Spinal dysraphism includes a broad category of malformations involving the dorsal midline aspect of the spine and spinal cord. These include findings of neural tube defects but can range to clinically silent anomalies. The various subtypes are named to specify the tissues types that are involved. For example, a meningocele contains dural layers without nerve tissue. Myelomeningocele will contain dural and neural elements. The major concern with these entities involves the potential of permanent neurologic deficits as well as ease of access for pathogens to enter the central nervous system.

The specific diagnosis is aided by CT or MRI. Findings include a dorsal midline defect within the spine and a posteriorly herniating sac into the subcutaneous tissues (Figure 15.9A and B). Based on CT density or MRI signal characteristics, the included components are determined. Most important, nerve involvement is discerned to aid in surgical management.[3,6]

## Caudal Regression

Caudal regression syndrome refers to a spectrum of congenital anomalies that deal with dysgenesis or even agenesis of the spine and spinal cord. Mild cases may be clinically silent; however, more severe cases result in major neurologic impairment of the gastrointestinal and genitourinary systems and lower extremities.

***Pearl:*** The incidence is significantly higher in children of diabetic mothers.

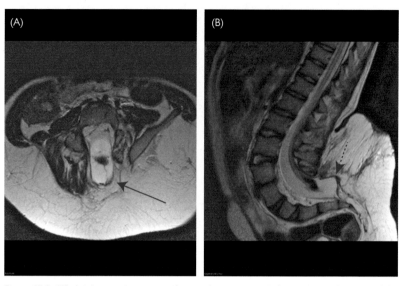

Figure 15.9 (**A**) Axial magnetic resonance image showing a gap in the posterior elements of the lower lumbar spine with herniation of the dural sac posteriorly (arrow 1). (**B**) Sagittal image of the same patient showing open communication of the spinal canal posteriorly into the subcutaneous fat of the lower back (arrow 2).

Diagnostic clues are most easily noted on MRI. It is identified by poorly or incompletely formed pelvis and distal vertebrae (Figure 15.10). Using sagittal images, the conus will appear blunted and/or foreshortened.[3,6]

## Pars Interarticularis Defect

Pars defects, otherwise known as spondylolysis, historically have had controversial underlying etiology. Most recently, however, they are believed to result from chronic, repetitive

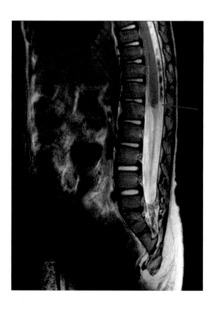

Figure 15.10 Sagittal magnetic resonance image showing a shortened cord with abrupt, blunted end at its distal margin (arrow). Additionally, note the segmental anomalies of the sacral spine.

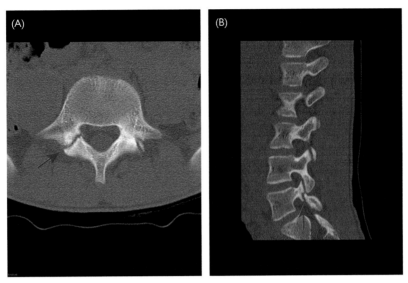

Figures 15.11 Axial (**A**) and sagittal (**B**) computed tomography images showing a linear lucency through the right pars of a lumbar vertebra (arrows). The margins are smooth and well corticated.

stress injury. These are most commonly seen at the L5 level, can be either unilateral or bilateral, and may be confused with acute fractures. While frequently asymptomatic, they can be a source of chronic pain. Larger concerns arise with development of spondylolisthesis, in which the involved vertebral levels may shift anteriorly or posteriorly relative to each other. This results in narrowing of the spinal canal and neural foramina and may lead to neurological impairment.

Diagnosis is most easily obtained with CT. Careful evaluation of the pars interarticularis is performed for a linear lucency similar to a fracture line (Figure 15.11A and B). The opposing portions of bone may develop a "pseudoarthrosis" due to bone-on-bone friction along the surfaces. Spondylolisthesis is identified on sagittal images by a vertebral body that appears as if it has translated anteriorly or posteriorly relative to adjacent levels.

### Ventriculus Terminalis

Ventriculus terminalis is sometimes called the "fifth ventricle." It is a congenital, benign fusiform dilatation of the central spinal canal near the conus. It is usually discovered as an incidental finding but is important to differentiate from a syrinx. Best seen on MRI, there will be mild fusiform expansion of the central spinal canal with no abnormal enhancement (Figure 15.12).

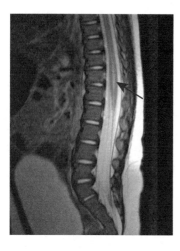

Figure 15.12 Sagittal magnetic resonance image of the spine shows subtle fusiform expansion of the central spinal canal (arrow) at the level of the conus.

# Brain

### Germinal Matrix Hemorrhage

The germinal matrix is a transient area (involutes late in the third trimester) with a rich vascular supply along the ependymal lining of the ventricles. This region acts a potential area of hemorrhage in response to perinatal stresses due to frailty and lack of central nervous system regulatory ability. Hemorrhage is seen in premature infants typically born before 32 weeks and can be screened and monitored with bedside sonography. A grading system is in place to help guide treatment and provide prognosis.

Ultrasound is the gold standard in evaluation because it is portable, fast, and accurate. Examination typically starts at the caudothalamic groove because this is the location for grade 1 hemorrhage. Additional evaluation is targeted to identify intraventricular hemorrhage, ventricular enlargement, and associated intraparenchymal hemorrhage because these findings elevate to grades 2, 3, and 4, respectively (Figure 15.13A–D).[2,7]

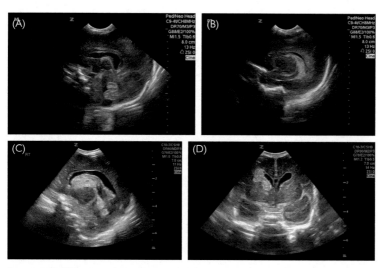

Figure 15.13 (**A**) Sagittal ultrasound image of a grade 1 hemorrhage with scant blood at the caudothalamic groove. (**B**) Sagittal ultrasound image of a grade 2 hemorrhage with blood products extending into the occipital horn. (**C**) Sagittal ultrasound image of a grade 3 hemorrhage with blood throughout the lateral ventricle with dilation of the ventricle. (**D**) Coronal ultrasound image of a grade 4 hemorrhage as blood extends out of the ventricles into the periventricular parenchyma.

## Periventricular Leukomalacia

Periventricular leukomalacia is the resultant finding after hypoxic-ischemic white-matter injury occurs perinatally, typically before 32 weeks' gestation. The white matter is highly susceptible during this time to inflammation from insult to immature oligodendrocytes. The irreparable damage can lead to volume loss and involution of the brain tissue. Changes of periventricular leukomalacia can be seen after high-grade germinal matrix hemorrhages.

Diagnosis is best made with ultrasound and MRI. Initially, white matter surrounding the lateral ventricles will appear brighter or more echogenic on ultrasound or have altered signal on MRI. After progression, these areas will cavitate and parenchyma will be replaced with cystic changes. The ventricles may enlarge from a vacuum effect related to parenchymal volume loss (Figure 15.14A and B).[2,7]

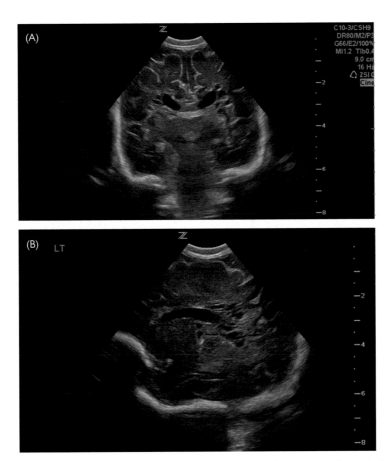

Figure 15.14 Coronal (**A**) and sagittal (**B**) ultrasound images showing cystic changes in the periventricular white matter, indicative of leukomalacia.

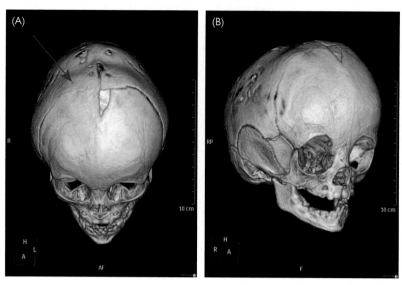

**Figures 15.15** (**A** and **B**) Three-dimensional reconstructed computed tomography images of a pediatric skull showing early fusion of the right coronal suture (arrow). Comparison can be made to the normal left coronal suture.

## Craniosynostosis

Craniosynostosis is a collection of skeletal abnormalities that result from abnormal early closure of a calvarial suture. As the calvarium continues to grow at the normal suture lines, asymmetry and distortion of the skull occurs, which can be seen on physical exam. Although these can occur sporadically, they can be congenital and syndromic in nature, potentiating the need for further medical evaluation.

Diagnosis exam can be made on physical exam; however, ultrasound and CT may be used to determine the sutures involved and to plan the surgical approach. The development of three-dimensional CT reformats is particularly useful, readily displaying the altered shape as well as the development of osseous or fibrous bridges.(Figure 15.15A and B).

## TORCH Infection

TORCH is an acronym for a set of pathogens that can cross the placenta and result in congenital infection. The acronym itself stands for T: toxoplasmosis, O: other (including HIV and syphilis), R: rubella, C: cytomegalovirus (CMV), and H: herpes. CMV infection is the most common of the organisms listed. Presentation will typically occur at birth or within the first few months of life, depending on the pathogen. Although there is an overlap in clinical and radiologic appearance, there are certain features that can help to identify the specific etiology.

Ultrasound, CT, and MRI each have a role in diagnosis. In general, TORCH infections will lead to injury of the periventricular white matter resulting in altered echogenicity, density, or signal (Figure 15.16A and B). CMV, toxoplasmosis, HIV, and rubella also may result in calcification. Herpes more frequently causes regions of hemorrhage to develop. CMV is best characterized by periventricular cysts and its ability to create migration abnormalities, which are discussed later.[2,8]

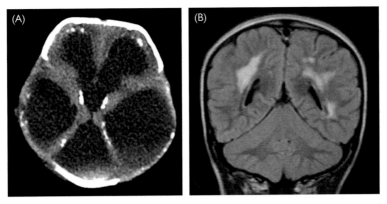

Figure 15.16 (**A**) Axial computed tomography showing dilated ventricles with small areas of periventricular calci-fication. (**B**) Coronal magnetic resonance image in a different patient showing altered signal in the periventricular white matter.

## Intracranial Tumors

Intra-axial (primary brain) tumors tend to have significant overlap in radiologic appearance leading to diagnostic uncertainty. They are best differentiated by age of the patient, location, and presence or absence of associated pathology. For the purposes of this chapter, the discussed intracranial tumors will be divided by typical location, including posterior fossa, supratentorial, intraventricular, and suprasellar.

### Posterior Fossa Neoplasms

Posterior fossa neoplasms include pilocytic astrocytoma, hemangioblastoma, ependymoma, medulloblastoma, and atypical teratoma/rhabdoid tumor. In posterior fossa masses, it is important to evaluate for an obstructing hydrocephalus because these tend to fill and/or compress the fourth ventricle. Additionally, there is a possibility of "drop metastases" requiring full imaging of the spine to assess for additional foci of the tumor.[2,9]

> **Pilocytic Astrocytoma.** Pilocytic astrocytoma is a World Health Organization (WHO) grade I tumor and is the most common primary brain tumor. It has an increased incidence in patients with neurofibromatosis type 1 (NF1) and typically arises from the cerebellum with compression of the fourth ventricle. It is seen on CT and MRI as a large cystic space with an enhancing mural nodule (Figure 15.17A and B).

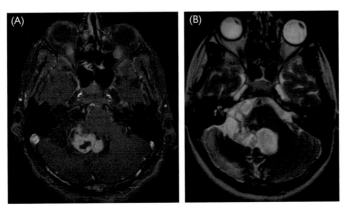

Figure 15.17 (**A** and **B**) Various axial magnetic resonance sequences showing a cystic mass in the posterior fossa with small, nodular solid component.

**Hemangioblastoma.** Hemangioblastoma is a WHO grade I tumor with high vascularity. It has an increased incidence in patients with von Hippel-Lindau syndrome. Imaging location and appearance is a cyst with an enhancing nodule, quite similar to a pilocytic astrocytoma. Hemangioblastomas tend to appear later in life, closer to adulthood (Figure 15.18A and B)

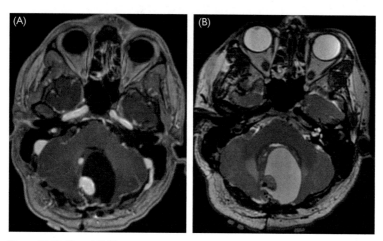

Figure 15.18 (**A** and **B**) Various magnetic resonance images at the level of the cerebellum showing a large, simple appearing cyst with enhancing nodule (arrow) along its medial wall.

**Ependymoma.** Ependymoma is a WHO grade II/III tumor based on histologic features. It is often described as a "plastic" or "toothpaste" tumor because of its ability to squeeze through spaces. CT and MRI will show a lobulated, solid tumor, which appears to arise within, and conform to, the fourth ventricle. The soft nature may show it extend through adjacent foramina.

**Medulloblastoma.** Medulloblastoma is a WHO grade IV tumor that is the most common malignant pediatric neoplasm and contains numerous subgroups. Similar to ependymoma, it will appear to arise from the fourth ventricle. It distinguishes itself from ependymoma by appearing more aggressive and invading adjacent structures, rather than extending through cerebrospinal fluid (CSF) spaces (Figure 15.19A and B).

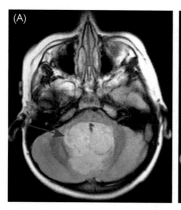
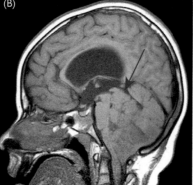

Figure 15.19 Axial (**A**) and sagittal (**B**) magnetic resonance images of an enhancing solid mass that fills and expands the fourth ventricle in the posterior fossa (arrows).

**Atypical Teratoma/Rhabdoid Tumor.** The atypical teratoma/rhabdoid tumor is a WHO grade IV tumor with poor prognosis. These tumors are highly aggressive and grow rapidly. On imaging, they are essentially indistinguishable from medulloblastoma. However, they have high cellular density, which can increase density on CT or show restricted diffusion on MRI.

## Supratentorial

Although supratentorial masses will have differentials based on radiologic appearance, certain features can favor a specific diagnosis. It is also important to evaluate the mass effect that occurs as supratentorial tumors may lead to hydrocephalus or herniation necessitating urgent intervention.

**Ganglioglioma.** Ganglioglioma is a WHO grade I/II tumor derived from ganglion and glial cells. The tumor is most notorious for being the etiology of temporal lobe epilepsy. On CT and MRI, it classically appears as a cystic mass with a solid enhancing component. Gangliogliomas are most frequently seen in the temporal lobe and can commonly have calcifications (Figure 15.20).

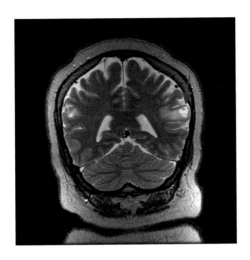

Figure 15.20 Coronal magnetic resonance image showing a small, multicystic mass in the left temporal lobe (arrows). Surrounding vasogenic edema is seen in the corresponding gyrus.

**DNET.** DNET is a WHO grade I tumor that has mixed glial and neuronal elements. Like the ganglioglioma, it favors the temporal lobe. Standard CT and MRI appearance is a "bubbly" multicystic mass. It less frequently contains calcification (Figure 15.21).

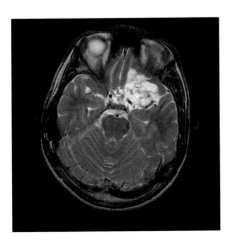

Figure 15.21 Axial magnetic resonance image demonstrating a "bubbly" cystic mass in the medial left temporal lobe.

**Pineoblastoma/Germinoma.** Pineoblastoma and germinoma are WHO grade II/III tumors affecting the pineal gland. The key to identification of pineal gland tumors is to know the location of the pineal gland. It sits at the midline, just inferior to the splenium of the corpus callosum. On CT and MRI there should be a mixed cystic/solid mass replacing the pineal gland (Figure 15.22). Due to mass effect on the tectal plate and sylvian aqueduct, there is a high potential for obstructive hydrocephalus.[2,3,9]

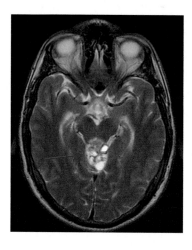

Figure 15.22 Axial magnetic resonance image with a midline, mixed cystic and solid mass in the expected location of the pineal gland (arrow).

*Pearl:* On CT, pineoblastomas and germinomas may be distinguished by their calcification patterns. Germinomas frequently show central calcification, whereas pineoblastomas are described as having "exploded" (peripheral) areas of calcification.

### Intraventricular

Unless identified incidentally, intraventricular tumors can remain clinically silent until considerable growth has occurred. This is because they have a relatively large, fluid-filled space to grow before imposing mass effect on adjacent structures.

**Choroid Plexus Tumors.** Choroid plexus tumors are WHO grade I/II/III tumors ranging from choroid plexus papilloma to carcinoma. Typically, these tumors will appear to arise and remain confined within the ventricles, although invasion into parenchyma can occur. On CT and MRI, there is a typical "cauliflower" appearance of an avidly enhancing mass. (Figure 15.23). Benign and malignant versions are essentially indistinguishable and treated similarly.

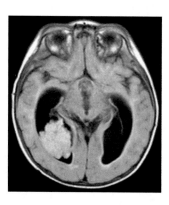

Figure 15.23 Axial magnetic resonance image with a "cauliflower" mass within the right lateral ventricle and associated hydrocephalus.

**Subependymal Giant Cell Astrocytoma (SEGA).** SEGA is a WHO grade I tumor. These tumors are relatively benign and slow growing and are seen almost exclusively in patients with tuberous sclerosis. The key in diagnosis is location. Classically, SEGA tumors will appear as brightly enhancing tumors at the foramen of Monro, which can lead to hydrocephalus of the affected lateral ventricle (Figure 15.24).

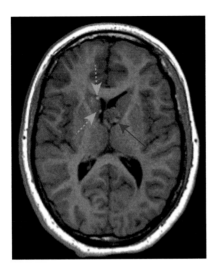

Figure 15.24 Axial magnetic resonance image showing a small, rounded mass situated at the left foramen of Monro (arrow 1). Small bright spots are seen at the subependymal lining of the right lateral ventricle (arrows 2), typical findings in a patient with tuberous sclerosis.

### Suprasellar

Suprasellar tumors are unique in their clinical presentation because of their location. The classic symptom is bitemporal hemianopsia due to the tumor's location just beneath the optic chiasm.

**Craniopharyngioma.** Craniopharyngioma is a WHO grade I tumor that arises from Rathke pouch. It has an excellent prognosis and curative potential with surgical excision. Best evaluation is with MRI identifying a predominantly cystic mass with enhancing components and calcification (Figure 15.25).

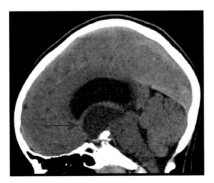

Figure 15.25 Sagittal computed tomography showing a large cystic mass in the suprasellar space (arrow) with calcification along the inferior margin.

**Hypothalamic Hamartoma.** Hypothalamic hamartoma is a congenital entity and is not truly neoplastic. Instead, it represents a disorganized focus of gray matter in the region of the tuber cinereum, which is bordered by the pons, mammillary bodies, and pituitary stalk (Figure 15.26). Clinically, it can result in precocious puberty and gelastic seizures, also known as laughing fits. On MRI, it will appear as a mass in the described location that will not enhance and will have signal characteristics nearly identical to gray matter.[2,3,9]

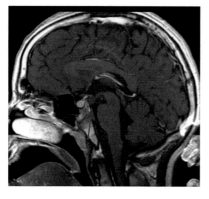

Figure 15.26 Sagittal magnetic resonance image demonstrating a small, rounded mass at the tuber cinereum (arrow) with signal features identical to gray matter.

## Leukodystrophies

Leukodystrophies are a category of congenital disorders that affect the ability to produce and preserve myelin. These are a result of various enzyme deficiencies that lead to specific diagnosis. Clinically, patients present with developmental deficiencies, which include behavioral difficulties, motor issues, and possibly seizures. Diagnosis is usually made with MRI. The typical pattern of myelination that occurs in the white matter is disrupted, causing altered low signal. The abnormalities occur in characteristic, symmetric locations (Figure 15.27). These different patterns help to differentiate subtypes. Magnetic resonance spectography is an additional tool used to measure cell turnover rates that supports diagnosis.

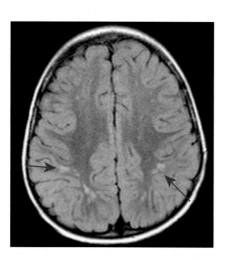

Figure 15.27 Axial magnetic resonance image showing symmetric foci of signal abnormality in the parietal lobe white matter (arrows). These features are suggestive of adrenoleukodystrophy.

## Trauma

Pediatric intracranial trauma is an unfortunate and all too common occurrence. The goal of imaging is to rapidly identify severity, evaluate for cases of nonaccidental trauma, and help guide management and intervention for the clinicians. The most common evidence of significant trauma is the identification of intracranial hemorrhage. Imaging is used for identification and localization of hemorrhage, evaluation of mass effect, and to look for associated edema of the brain parenchyma.[1,2,7]

### Epidural Hematoma

An epidural hematoma, commonly associated with a fracture, occurs when blood accumulates beneath the skull, superficial to the dura. Epidural hematomas tend to be arterial in origin (middle meningeal artery) and can have significant mass effect. CT and MRI will demonstrate a biconvex accumulation of hyperdense blood that is contained within the boundaries of the calvarial sutures (Figure 15.28).

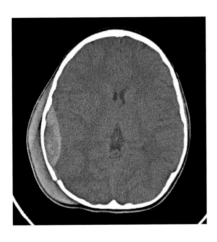

Figure 15.28 Axial computed tomography showing a hyperdense collection of blood in the epidural space along the right frontoparietal lobe. Additional findings include a fracture in the parietal calvarium as well as overlying scalp hematoma.

### Subdural Hematoma

A subdural hematoma is blood that accumulates between the dura and arachnoid spaces. Subdural hematomas tend to develop at a slower rate than epidural hematomas and should be monitored. CT and MRI will demonstrate a crescent-shaped hyperdense collection of blood that will cross suture boundaries but will not cross midline at the anterior-posterior aspects of the skull (Figure 15.29).

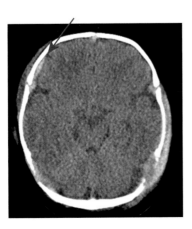

Figure 15.29 Axial computed tomography showing a thin, crescent-shaped collection of blood along the right frontal lobe (arrow).

## Subarachnoid Hemorrhage

A subarachnoid hemorrhage occurs when blood accumulates beneath the arachnoid membrane and above the pia mater. CT and MRI will show blood accumulation within CSF spaces, including sulci, cisterns, and ventricles (Figure 15.30). It is important to identify a subarachnoid hemorrhage because coagulated blood can negatively affect arachnoid granulations, which may lead to hydrocephalus.

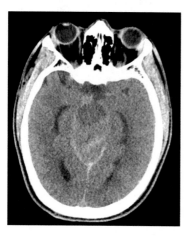

Figure 15.30 Axial computed tomography showing hyperdense blood within the ambient and perimesencephalic cisterns.

## Vascular Malformations

Intracranial vascular malformations can be congenital or sporadic manifestations. The term *vascular malformation* is a "wastebasket" term that can include multiple types of anomalies. Many of these are incidentally noted during intracranial imaging for other purposes. Symptoms arise if they become unusually large or hemorrhage. Four categories of malformation are briefly discussed here.

## Arteriovenous Malformation

Arteriovenous malformations are an abnormal communication of arterioles and venules without a capillary bed. They have a specific grading system that is used to determine whether intervention is recommended. Most have low risk for hemorrhage. CT angiography or magnetic resonance angiography will show an enhancing tangle of arteries at a nidus, typically with a prominent draining vein (Figure 15.31). The disruptive flow can lead to calcification.

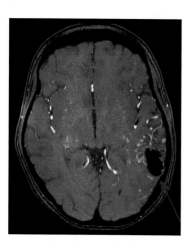

Figure 15.31 Axial magnetic resonance image showing a tangle of vessels in the left parietal lobe. Globular area of low signal (arrow) indicates regions of calcification.

## Cavernous Malformation (Cavernoma)

A cavernoma is thought to be a result of microscopic hemorrhage that leads to angiogenesis, resulting in thin, immature vessels. It can be congenital and have an association with developmental venous anomaly (DVA). CT and MRI will show a typical "popcorn" appearance of calcification in a localized lesion (Figure 15.32). No distinct abnormal vessels are seen, even with angiographic imaging.

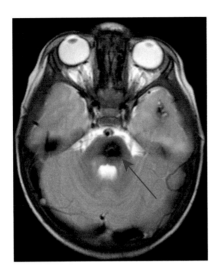

Figure 15.32 Axial magnetic resonance image with region of popcorn calcification within the pons (arrow) and no surrounding abnormal vessels.

## Developmental Venous Anomaly

A DVA is frequently an incidental finding consisting of mature veins. It is sometimes considered to be a normal anatomic variant. Contrast enhanced CT or MRI will reveal a characteristic "Medusa head" of prominent veins that drain into a single prominent vein (Figure 15.33).

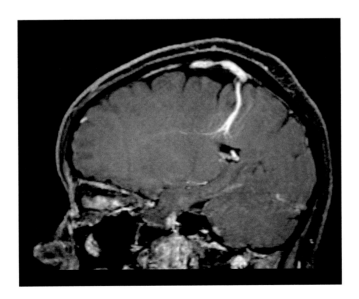

Figure 15.33 Sagittal magnetic resonance image demonstrating a prominent vein in the parietal region draining toward the cortex.

**15.** Pediatric Neurologic Radiology

## Capillary Telangiectasia

Capillary telangiectasia is a small collection of abnormal, dilated capillaries. This condition can be seen in association with other vascular malformations. Unlike other malformations, telangiectases more frequently occur in the posterior fossa, brainstem, and spine. They tend to be occult on CT and MRI, but contrast imaging may show a focused blush of contrast.

## Moyamoya

This vascular entity is present as both a primary inherited disorder and a secondary process to systemic diseases that result in arterial injury and pathology. Sickle cell disease is a common underlying factor. Regardless of etiology, the result is severe narrowing or occlusion of the internal carotid arteries and circle of Willis. This results in the formation of numerous, fragile collateral vessels that tend to be insufficient. Clinical manifestations are from the resultant transient ischemic attacks that occur.[2,3]

CT angiography and magnetic resonance angiography are used to carefully evaluate the distal portions of the internal carotid arteries. The affected arteries will be significantly narrowed or occluded. There will be an adjacent complex network of small collateral vessels that intervene through parenchyma (Figure 15.34A and B) MRI is also useful to identify areas of acute ischemia.

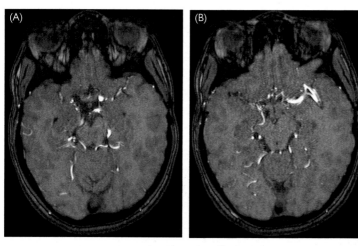

**Figure 15.34 (A and B)** Axial magnetic resonance angiograms showing a diminutive right middle cerebral artery at the level of the suprasellar cistern and sylvian fissure. Comparison can be made to the normal left side.

## Dandy-Walker Malformation

Dandy-Walker malformation is frequently a sporadic occurrence but is also associated with congenital syndromes and other fetal anomalies. It occurs from interrupted development of the cerebellar vermis. The diagnosis is now frequently made in utero during screening exams but can present with delayed development or secondary symptoms from resulting hydrocephalus. Although seen on ultrasound, MRI is more useful for complete evaluation and differentiation from similar entities. There will be a partial or complete midline defect of the cerebellum (vermis) with cyst-like expansion of the fourth ventricle and posterior fossa

(Figure 15.35). The mass effect can displace the tentorium superiorly and impress on the brainstem, which is best appreciated on sagittal views.[2,3]

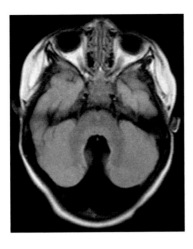

**Figure 15.35** Axial magnetic resonance image with a midline cleft and defect of the cerebellum where the vermis normally resides.

### Migration and Proliferation Anomalies

Because of the complex orchestration of central nervous system development, there are many anomalous manifestations that can occur within the brain due to arrest or disorganization of neuronal migration and development. The etiology is not always clear but can range from sporadic occurrence to congenital associations and maternal factors during pregnancy. Although frequently discovered on screening ultrasound, clinical features include delays in sensory-motor skills, behavioral abnormalities, seizures, and cranial nerve deficiencies.[2,3]

### Schizencephaly

Schizencephaly is an example of neuronal migration error or potential microvascular injury. MRI will show a defect or cleft that extends the ventricles to the cortical surface and is lined with gray matter (Figure 15.36). Schizencephaly is described as being "open lipped" or "closed lipped" depending on the presence or absence of CSF within the defect.

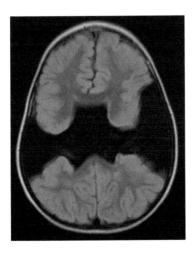

**Figure 15.36** Axial magnetic resonance image showing direct communication from the lateral ventricles to the cortex through symmetric, open lip clefts.

***Pearl:*** The presence of gray matter lining the cleft is helpful in differentiating schizencephaly from a porencephalic cyst, which can extend to the brain surface but will not be lined by gray matter.

## Gray Matter Heterotopia

Gray matter heterotopia is a neuronal migration error resulting in focal or laminar distributions of gray matter outside of the cerebral cortex. MRI best demonstrates the ectopic or heterotopic gray matter. The most common location is along the ependymal lining of the ventricles (Figure 15.37). The abnormal areas will follow signal characteristics of the cortex.

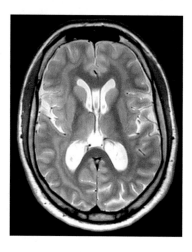

**Figure 15.37** Axial magnetic resonance image demonstrating abnormally distributed gray matter surrounding the lateral ventricles.

## Lissencephaly

A spectrum of findings are associated with lissencephaly because it can be an isolated entity or part of a larger syndrome. The defining characteristic on imaging is a smooth cortical surface. This can be seen with abnormally small, large, or absent gyri (Figure 15.38). Of note, this can be incorrectly diagnosed if the gestational age is inaccurate.

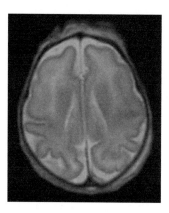

**Figure 15.38** Axial magnetic resonance image revealing a distinct lack of sulci resulting in a smooth, lobular cortical surface.

The last four diagnoses to be discussed are best explained together owing to the similar imaging features, despite having different etiologies. The presence or absence of certain intracranial structures will help to make the correct diagnosis.

## Hydrocephalus

Hydrocephalus is a generic term used to describe abnormal enlargement of the ventricles from overabundant CSF. Massive hydrocephalus can fill nearly the entire cranium and significantly displace brain parenchyma peripherally. On ultrasound, CT, and MRI, there will be significantly enlarged ventricles. The key is to identify residual, thinned parenchyma that has been displaced to the calvarial inner table and the presence of a falx cerebri (Figure 15.39).[2,3]

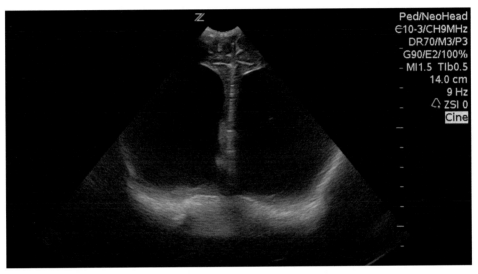

**Figure 15.39** Coronal ultrasound image with massively dilated lateral ventricles. It is important to note the presence of falx cerebri at the midline and residual cortical tissue along the periphery.

## Hydranencephaly

Hydranencephaly results in utero from vascular compromise of the anterior circulation. This causes complete lack of development of the cerebral hemispheres and fluid replacement (Figure 15.40), but the posterior fossa and dura are intact. Differentiation from hydrocephalus is made by the lack of cortical mantle (peripheral, thinned parenchyma), and the presence of the falx cerebri will also distinguish it from other entities.[2,3]

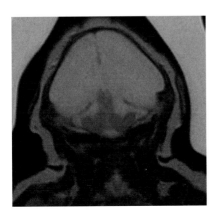

**Figure 15.40** Coronal magnetic resonance image with distinct lack of supratentorial brain tissue. The dura remain intact in addition to posterior fossa elements.

## Holoprosencephaly (Alobar)

Holoprosencephaly has a spectrum of severity. For simplicity, alobar will be described because it has more pronounced features. The pathology results after failure of midline cleavage of the cerebral hemispheres and midline structures. This can result in a single, enlarged "monoventricle" that mimics the entities described previously (Figure 15.41). To differentiate, with alobar there will be a lack of the midline structures such as the falx cerebri. There will be fused thalami and some intact cortical brain tissue.[2,3,6]

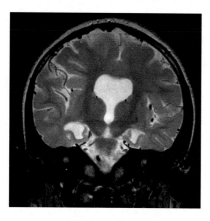

Figure 15.41 Coronal magnetic resonance image showing a single, monoventricle lacking a septum. The falx is absent.

## Anencephaly

The most severe manifestation of this group, anencephaly is the end result of an open neural tube defect in which the skull does not properly form. The exposed brain tissue is destroyed in utero, leading to complete absence of normal brain above the brainstem. There will be a fluid-filled cartilaginous cranium, similar to the diagnoses described previously. However, owing to lack of structural support elements, the calvarium will be flattened or collapsed with exposed residual neural tissue (Figure 15.42).[2,3,6]

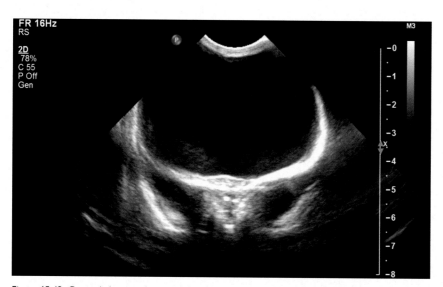

Figure 15.42 Coronal ultrasound image with intracranial contents completely replaced with fluid. The superior calvarium is also collapsed and concave because it lacks structural elements.

# References

1. Burrow TA, Saal HM, de Alarcon A, et al. Characterization of congenital anomalies in individuals with choanal atresia. *Arch Otolaryngol Head Neck Surg.* 2009;135(6):543–547.

2. Osborn A, Jhaveri MD, Salzman KL, Barkovich AJ. *Diagnostic Imaging: Brain.* 1st ed. Salt Lake City: Amirsys; 2004.

3. Barkovich A, Raybaud C. *Pediatric Neuroimaging.* 3rd ed. Philadelphia: Lippincott-Raven; 2000.

4. Benson MT, Dalen K, Mancuso AA, et al. Congenital anomalies of the branchial apparatus: embryology and pathologic anatomy. *Radiographics.* 1992;12(5):943–960.

5. Tateishi U, Hasegawa T, Miyakawa K, et al. CT and MRI features of recurrent tumors and second primary neoplasms in pediatric patients with retinoblastoma. *AJR Am J Roentgenol.* 2003;181(3):879–884.

6. Wilson RD; SOGC Genetics Committee; Special Contributor. Prenatal screening, diagnosis, and management of fetal neural tube defects. *J Obstet Gynaecol.* 2014;36(10):927–939.

7. Blankenberg FG, Loh NN, Bracci P, et al. Sonography, CT, and MR imaging: a prospective comparison of neonates with suspected intracranial ischemia and hemorrhage. *AJNR Am J Neuroradiol.* 2000;21(1)213–218.

8. Nickerson JP, Richner B, Santy K, et al. Neuroimaging of pediatric intracranial infection—part 2: TORCH, viral, fungal and parasitic infections. *J Neuroimaging.* 2012;22(2):52–63.

9. Hwang SW, Su JM, Jea A. Diagnosis and management of brain and spinal cord tumors in the neonate. *Semin Fetal Neonatal Med.* 2012;17(4):202–206.

**15.** Pediatric Neurologic Radiology

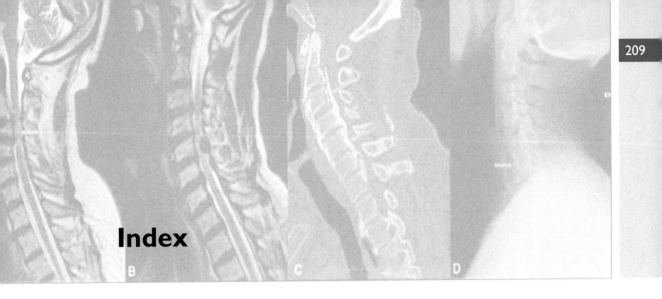

# Index

Tables and figures are indicated by *t* and *f* following the page number